The 7 Seven Initiations of the Spiritual Path

by Michael Mirdad

D1024113

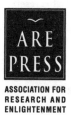

ARE PRESS

ASSOCIATION FOR
RESEARCH AND
ENLIGHTENMENT

A.R.E. Press • Virginia Beach • Virginia

A.R.E. Press
215 67th Street
Virginia Beach, VA 23451-2061

Library of Congress Control Number: 2004302022

Cover design by Richard Boyle

Contents

How It Looks
The Dark Night of the Soul
You Are Unique
Mysteries of the Heart
The Limitations of the Heart
The Gifts of the Heart
Modern Parallels
Facets of the Heart and Soul–Air

How It Looks
Accepting Your Divinity
Every Day Is Christmas
The Limits of Spirit
The Gifts of the Spirit
Modern Parallels
Facets of the Spirit–Ether

How It Looks
Inner Peace Before Outer Peace
Integration Means Immunity
The Divine Feminine

How It Looks
God Recycles
Why We Keep Coming Back
Ascended Masters: The Exception to the Rule

In the End, There Is a Purpose After All
Conclusion

Acknowledgments

I extend my deepest appreciation to all those individuals who have assisted in the manifestation of this book and to everyone (friends, students, clients, tour sponsors, etc.) who has supported my teachings over the greater part of my life. I thank Brian Smith, Mark Ortman, and "The Three Sisters"—Cassandra, Christian, and Krystall. I also thank Robin Rose (one of my dearest soulmates) for coordinating the annual Universal Lightworkers Conference and letting me be a part. There is no other event like it! Last, but not least, this book is also dedicated to all of God's children who have endured the "dark night of the soul" and sought the "light at the end of the tunnel."

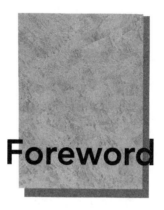

Foreword

Like everyone else, you have experienced tumultuous changes while navigating the rites of passage of your life. These changes have produced a range of intense reactions within you—sometimes enticing you forward with love, sometimes scarring and immobilizing you with fear. Some of your experiences involved joy, even ecstasy—an ineffable and soaring transfiguration of the heart. Other experiences kindled a searing and unbearable pain whose final traces smolder to this day—deep within.

At times you felt as though you were glimpsing something of the deeper purpose behind your major changes. At other times you were dashed upon the rocks of confusion and despair. But you have always felt inexorably compelled to seek an ever-deepening understanding of the true significance behind your great turning points.

The initiations of my own life burn within me to this day. Many of them are similar in essence to your own. I remember as a teenager watching my father die alone before me on a mountaintop in Vermont one spring day, and I remember administering CPR until a physician arrived at the scene and pronounced him dead—and I remember as the eldest having to tell my mother.

I vividly recall when I fell head–over–heels in love for the first time, and I remember when my heart was broken so badly that I could not think straight for a year. I remember when, in my early twenties, alcohol and drugs brought me to my knees, and I recall with wonder and gratitude the miraculous process of recovery that occurred when I surrendered to a power greater than myself and accepted its help and guidance. I remember when my body's kundalini energy rose for the first time and all the hair on my body stood on end as I meditated in a corn field one dazzling fall day.

There were the intense book camps of medical school and internship, an office embezzlement, wealth, bankruptcy, marriage, the birth of my son, a spiritual divorce, and the publication of my first book.

We all have our own intense turning points, our own momentous enlightenments, and our own crushing tragedies. No one is exempt. Even Christ and Buddha enjoyed and endured the classic initiations that life on this planet inevitably places before us. Our passage through these sometimes thundering rapids are the most important things that ever happen for us. These experiences hammer and forge our souls. They stamp our hearts and minds with the indelible imprint of Spirit. And, pleasant or agonizing, they provide unerring corrections on our paths to love, our paths to God.

As you read the book that follows, you will recall your own great milestones, and you will perceive them no longer through a glass darkly but with new eyes—as though illuminated with a clear and powerful light. Your mind will be opened, your heart released, and your spirit expanded far beyond their ordinary boundaries. As you contemplate the words that follow, you will finally understand—with unprecedented clarity—the *true* meaning of your tragedies and your successes.

In truth, for many of you, the very reading of this groundbreaking book will provide yet another important initiation. Pay careful attention. For my friend and colleague, Dr. Michael Mirdad, is an ancient soul with a profound wealth of light and knowledge. If you will trust his intent and open to his wisdom and expertise, the chapters that follow will catapult you to a new, quantum level of energy and understanding. Namaste,

Dr. Michael Abrams
Author of the bestseller *The Evolution Angel* and *The Twelve Conditions of a Miracle—The Miracle Worker's Handbook.*

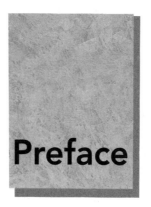

Preface

I feel as if I've been aware of how things work here on earth, from a spiritual perspective, for most of my life. Like many students of spirituality, I've always felt I was different from most other people. Growing up, I was not sure how to get the answers to the numerous questions that filled my mind. Often, when I asked family or friends, I only received raised eyebrows. Yet, this lack of response and support in my childhood led me on a search that resulted in my having to "go within" to get answers. Here I found God, love, support, and Divine Guidance.

In junior high (middle school), I had only a few friends in whom I could confide my intuitive/mystical awarenesses and insights, and even *they* had mixed responses. Yet, by the time I reached high school, I was getting a clear picture of life—its patterns, purpose, and meaning. Eventually, parents started sending their children (my friends) to me for counseling through their rough times. I later found that experiences similar to mine were common among "Lightworkers" or students of the spiritual path.

After graduating from high school, like many eighteen year olds, I was terrified at the thought of what my future might hold. What was I going to do with my life? The career counselors asked me about my interests. I only knew that I liked people and wanted to improve their lives. I was advised that this was a nice sentiment but hardly a realistic way to make a good living. So, I registered for college, primarily to avoid the onslaught of family pressure to get a "real job." There, I focused on the courses related to health and psychology. By this time, I was also deeply immersed in the work of Edgar Cayce and the teachings of *A Course in Miracles*.

Shortly afterward, I was fortunate enough to stumble upon one of the many schools of metaphysics in southern California. I enrolled in spiritual classes by night, while attending college by day. On weekends, I went to every healing workshop I could find. Before long, all of these pieces of my education merged and became a large part of my life. By the time I was in my early twenties, I had a diverse background in psychology and numerous healing arts, as well as a doctorate in metaphysics. Even before I had completed my studies, I had begun teaching private classes on a wide variety of subjects, ranging, for example, from Atlantis and angels to relationships and sexuality.

My teaching and counseling career began over twenty years ago. Since then, I have been blessed with the gift of finding and living my *soul's purpose*—teaching workshops and offering private sessions. Furthermore, I have made a living doing what I enjoy most, while also touching the lives of others.

Along the way, however, without warning, LIFE HAPPENED! One of the great tests that befalls us individually, commonly referred to as the "dark night of the soul," paid me a visit. After losing most, or all, of the things I valued, I learned that the true purpose of this dark night is to encourage us to open our hearts, live in balance (heart, mind, feelings, and body), practice the art of surrender to God, and integrate all we have learned and experienced. I also learned that the dark night of the soul is simply one of life's major initiations into the next level of awareness.

By this time in my life, I had come to understand that each of life's tests/initiations correlates to one of our primary states of consciousness (chakras, or spiritual centers). In other words, all of life's tests are simply the calling of the soul, via our spiritual centers, to move forward. We always respond to this calling. We either hear it and follow, or we try to deny (or at least alter) the call in a way that brings the lessons of initiation in a more dramatic/traumatic way. This book is about how to recognize and heed these growth impulses from the soul. It also reminds us that all roads *do* eventually lead home—to a heavenlike state of consciousness. Thank God!

> *Hope is the eternal light held aloft by the soul as man travels the pathway . . . to reach God.*
>
> —**Paramahansa Yogananda**

Part I

Introduction

GETTING STARTED

After twenty years of teaching workshops related to the theme of this book, I knew it was time to finally share this information in book form. The workshops were originally a compilation of personal experiences, as well as information from the numerous classes I had facilitated on such topics as healing the human energy systems, initiations, ancient civilizations, and spirituality.

This book, therefore, is the culmination of extensive study, application (internal and external), and teaching of the various topics that usually pave the path to spiritual growth. I'm certain you will find that the material is diverse enough to appeal to beginners as well as advanced students of spirituality. Everyone will probably relate well to the material because everyone (consciously or not) walks the path of spirituality.

Therefore, it can be used as a wonderful map and a valuable guide for all who embark on "THE SPIRITUAL PATH."

Although this book contains widely accepted concepts and supporting quotes and cross-references, it is still subject to each person's interpretation. Your own experiences along the spiritual path may differ in varying degrees. Also, as you read, remember to maintain a sense of humor. Like the legendary mystic Dante, who refers to our experiences in the universe as the "Divine Comedy," it is my teaching style to keep things light.

It is highly recommended that rather than merely *reading* this book, allow it to be experienced. Let this experience be a dialogue between you and your higher self. In other words, instead of letting your intellectual mind browse through the material with its usual curiosity, allow yourself to digest, integrate, and apply what is written and shared. If you let go, you will find that the material in this book seems organic and natural to your soul. This is the way truth feels.

Finally, to better understand the material found in this book and to avoid confusion with various thought systems, let's take a moment to clarify some terminology—especially since many people use several spiritually related words interchangeably.

INITIATIONS AND LIFE'S TESTS

There are a total of seven major initiations that all human beings experience on their journeys toward wholeness. Initiations can be referred to as "life tests" or "spiritual tests" that are placed in our path for our soul's growth. These tests do not occur only once, but instead recycle around and around, bringing us to higher levels of awareness. We are always going through initiations, whether we are conscious of it or not. However, becoming conscious of these tests offers a quantum leap forward on our evolutionary journey.

TWO PATHS FOR ALL

There are actually *two* paths related to personal growth. One is commonly referred to as *THE SPIRITUAL PATH*. The other is

THE HEALING PATH. Some Native American traditions refer to these two paths as that of Father–Wisdom and Mother–Healing. The great symbol of the caduceus represents (among other things) these two paths connecting each state of human consciousness to the Consciousness of the Divine. To live in balance and attain mastery and wholeness, *both* of these paths must be equally embraced and nurtured.

Therefore, placing extra emphasis on the spiritual path (and neglecting the healing path) often results in a person who reads, prays, meditates, practices a religion or complex philosophical system, but spends little time nurturing the body or accessing and healing emotional issues.

On the other hand, placing extra emphasis on the healing path (with far less focus on the spiritual path) usually manifests as a person who does yoga or tai chi, observes nutritional laws, exercises, is very earth conscious, does breathwork, or nurtures the "inner child," but tends to neglect spiritual practices.

CADUCEUS AND THE TWO PATHS TO WHOLENESS

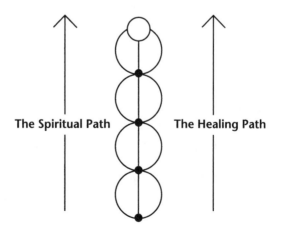

The Spiritual Path   The Healing Path

SPIRIT, SOUL, AND BODY

In this book, the term *Spirit* is usually capitalized because it denotes our true divine identity. God is Spirit and, being created in God's image, we too are Spirit.

The term *soul* (which is synonymous with our "higher mind" and is found in our heart center) is used to indicate the new identity we took on *after* we seemed to have separated from God and, therefore, from our true identity. The soul is synonymous with the heart and is that part of us that lives beyond the life span of the body, journeying in and out of the lower realms of manifestation—on an evolutionary path.

Finally, the term *body* indicates the physical and emotional self, as well as what is commonly referred to as the "lower (intellectual) mind." **When the opportunities for learning lessons in a particular life are completed, the body dies, and the soul moves on into higher realms until it needs to return again for other lessons or initiations.**

> *Our body is from the very beginning a mandala. Our state of consciousness is from the beginning, spirit. When one has entered into this knowledge of that which one is, then one is what one is, and that is what we call true initiation.* —*Araga, Tibetan Master*

When all lessons are learned, the soul (like the body) will also surrender its existence and merge back into its originating Spirit and oneness with God. This process is described in the introduction of *The Aquarian Gospel of Jesus the Christ*, by Levi, as follows: "The Spirit . . . is one with God . . . and cannot die. When man has conquered every foe [test] upon the plane of soul . . . the garb of soul will then have served its purpose well, and man will need it never more, and it will pass and be no more." This process of the soul returning to its Source is also described in the Book of Revelation where it speaks of a wedding, or merging, between a bride (the soul) and a Divine bridegroom (the Divine Self, Christ, or God).

CHAKRAS, SPIRITUAL CENTERS, AND INITIATIONS

Most students on the spiritual path are familiar with the term *chakra*. However, it's important to clarify the definition and symbolism in the context of the material in this book.

The word *chakra* is ancient Sanskrit and means "spinning wheel" or "vortex." Vortexes, or chakras, are also known as "spiritual centers" of energy and consciousness. It is commonly believed that there are seven *major* chakras within the body that correspond to seven major endocrine glands (for example, the pituitary, adrenals, and thymus). These vortexes of energy emerge to the surface on the front and back of the body from seven regions of the spine that correlate to the endocrine glands. The seven major initiations we all experience in life relate to one or more of these centers because **each chakra represents a different state of consciousness—relevant to our journey toward wholeness.**

Most schools of thought agree with the spiritual significance of the upper three centers and the meaning of the heart center. However, there is often confusion and disagreement among thought systems as to which centers correspond to which aspects of consciousness in the three anatomically lower centers. There are discrepancies as to which of the three lower centers relates to the physical, emotional, and mental aspects of human consciousness. The material in this book views the body as a map for gaining greater clarity as to a person's place on the path of evolution. On this symbolic map of the body, the three upper centers (chakras) correspond to the Divine Trinity and our Spiritual Divinity. The four lower centers (chakras) located in the torso are attributed to standard archetypes of the four states of consciousness—physical, emotional, mental, and intuitive.

In actuality, the first two lower centers (root and navel) are very much related to physical life and being. The second and third centers (navel and solar plexus) are primarily emotional centers, and the third and fourth centers (solar plexus and heart) are commonly seen as relating to the mind. If you remember this, it will help to alleviate any confusion as to which centers correlate to which aspects of consciousness, especially when you encounter discrepancies in various materials and thought systems. In other words, when seen in the light of the above explanation, all of the diverse versions are valid. However, they each approach the subject from a different angle.

TWO VERSIONS OF THE CHAKRAS AS A KEY

Spiritual Centers	(○ ○ ○)	(○ ○ ○) Spiritual Centers
Intuitive Center	○	○ ⎱ Mental Centers
Mental Center	○	○ ⎰
		Emotional Centers
Emotional Center	○	○
		Physical Centers
Physical Center	○	○

THE MEANING OF CHRIST

The name *Christ* might be the most important term or word to clarify, as it is occasionally used throughout this book. First of all, there should be no confusion between the terms "Christ Consciousness" and "Christianity." The first refers to the state of consciousness that Jesus attained. The latter refers to the organized religion with which Jesus had little or nothing to do.

The term *Christ* is pre-Christian and means "the True Self of *all* of God's children." All who remember their Identity in God become the Christ. So, Jesus might best be referred to as "Jesus, who remembered he is Christ," or "Jesus the Christ." **The yearning to remember who we really are is the motivation behind everything else we seek and experience.**

> *Let the Christ mind that was born in Jesus, be born in you as well.* — The Bible (Philippians 2:5)

Part II

The Journey Begins

Part II discusses how the "spiritual path" began and introduces the two roads of traveling on the spiritual path—the easy way and the hard way. This section also reviews the symbolism of initiations and relates these initiations to our lives and our life-lessons. It is advisable that you read the Introduction before proceeding any further. Also, if any parts of the book do not seem clear, just keep reading, as you may find greater clarification soon follows.

The first chapter in this section reviews the concept of our true, eternal Identity—our Spirit—as well as our false, temporary self—the evolving soul.

The second and third chapters review the history and significance of initiations in ancient and modern civilizations. Here, the esoteric meaning of geometry, numbers, and symbols is also introduced.

There are times in this section (and throughout the book) when initiations are referred to as one gradual procession we evolve through—over many lifetimes. However, at other times, it will appear that initiations occur on a daily basis and/or during certain periods of our lives. Although it may sound like a contradiction, both of these views are true. The former refers to initiations in the "macrocosmic" sense (the big picture). The latter depicts initiations in the "microcosmic" sense (the baby steps, or mini-initiations of life).

A good example of the mutual validity of this apparent contradiction is evident in people who have major issues with abandonment. They might be processing this issue throughout their entire lives—or many lifetimes (macrocosm). Yet, they might also deal with large and small individual segments, or aspects, of abandonment several times per day or per year (microcosm).

Both of these levels of initiation (macrocosm and microcosm) are equally valid and essential. The fundamental difference is that microcosmic initiations are like smaller, spinning wheels that revolve many times to gradually allow the single, larger wheel to turn once. Again, both are vital; but the one, greater evolution of life is totally dependent on the progress of the smaller, day-to-day and moment-by-moment accomplishments. These are like cycles within cycles that take the form of smaller lessons assisting in learning larger lessons.

The last chapter in this section (Chapter 4) reviews how we *seem* to have separated from our original Source—God—how we re-created ourselves and took on a lesser identity—the evolving soul—and how the soul has refracted its experience into four distinct facets of consciousness to understand itself and for use as a map to review its progress. This last chapter closes with a review of what each of the four levels of initiation involves and offers my own experiences of these tests.

1

The Spiritual Path

Do you remember when you embarked on your spiritual path? For most people, this turning point is like going into recovery, not from drugs or alcohol, but from "life" itself. Therefore, they identify the beginning of their spiritual journey with a time frame wherein the choice was made to become more conscious and responsible for their journey or to follow some form of spiritual discipline.

> *When one realizes one is asleep, at that moment one is already half awake.* —Ouspensky and Gurdjieff

The truth is, we all have an indwelling **spirit**. This means that every **path** we have ever walked was, and is, a **spiritual path**. In fact, the word *spiritual* is a combination of the words *spirit* and *ritual*. So, it could be said that our spiritual path is a journey filled with rituals or initiations. Sure, we may not have realized it. In fact, there are probably numerous deeds and experiences we are *unlikely* to refer to as part of our "spiritual path." Nevertheless, **no matter what paths we've walked or roads we've chosen, because our spirit was present, they were all spiritual paths. There are no exceptions!**

To know the universe itself as a road, as many roads, roads for traveling souls. — Walt Whitman

IT'S ALL GOOD—ALL PATHS LEAD HOME

The idea of spiritual evolution makes great sense and is reasonable because it assures a good chance of learning—at various levels. Yet, the theory of evolution conceals an ego concept that claims we have lots of work to do, to make better that which God made perfect in the first place. So we learn to believe the only way we can earn our way back home is to work hard to *perfect* all aspects of ourselves until we reach wholeness, a task which, I might add, holds little chance. The problem with this theory of evolution is that the universe takes our thoughts very literally. So, **if we believe we have work to do, it means we believe we are not already perfect, which means we have stepped outside of God's Consciousness.** Once we separate, we are outside of perfection (or at least seem to be). We will then attract all kinds of experiences that will reflect our beliefs back to us—beliefs of being separate and having work to do.

The good news, however, is that if you have invested a great deal of time working on yourself, usually you will catch on. You will realize this drive to *perfect* yourself was all a game, because the very thing you were searching for was within you all along—your true, Divine Self. Yet, not everyone catches on right away. Some people get so overwhelmed by the many choices along the path of spiritual growth they become distracted by (or even stuck in) some form of dogma or perhaps by working too hard to reach a wholeness that is already theirs at the accepting. One of the best ways to escape this trap is to recognize that a common theme runs throughout all aspects of the spiritual path. **All paths are actually just different perspectives of the same Truth and**

will ultimately lead to God.

Love has no opposite, but it does have opposition.
                                          —Jerry Bartholow

You may have spent some time in your life exploring or experimenting with sex and drugs, or celibacy and organic living. Whichever the case, **all choices are equally an attempt by the soul to learn lessons and explore itself and its environment.** From this viewpoint, it is possible to look at people, the world, and the choices we or others have made and see that the judgments are neither necessary nor valuable. All choices ultimately play a part in our growth; all roads lead home!

It's almost impossible to go through the numerous forms of this earthly experience and spiritual searching without realizing that you *are* connected to God. But you can, however, block God out of your life and conscious awareness to a point where you doubt or deny God's existence. You can become a great archer, a financial whiz or master some other field—even *without* a conscious connection with God. On the other hand, you can also do it *with* God. Doing it without God leading the way is simply trying to do it the hard way, even though all roads still lead home—to the awareness of God. It's just that the hard path takes much more time and potentially involves more pain. This longer path (the one without God) also includes what some thought systems refer to as the seemingly endless cycle of karma.

Regardless of which path we choose, all of the various states of consciousness found within the human psyche are of equal importance. The heart center might *seem* to play a higher role than the root, physical center, but they are all equally valuable to our growth or remembrance process.

Again, one state of consciousness is not *better* than another. A heart-focused Buddhist is not superior to an earth-focused Wiccan. They *all* represent a part of our evolution. One is simply more heart-based, while the other is more earth-based. In fact, from the perspective of Spirit, there is no separation, nor difference, between these two states of consciousness or any other. For example, **it will never serve you well to**

claim to have a "heart-based consciousness" and yet have a condescending attitude toward someone who is more physical or health centered. Even being heart centered has potential pitfalls, such as an unhealthy detachment from the world and excessive denial. There are many individuals whose lives suffer because they believe themselves to be more "spiritual" than everyone else. It always leads to trouble whenever one path, which only represents *one* of several states of human consciousness, is considered to be superior to all others. This reasoning makes as much sense as your stomach claiming to be greater than your liver. Of course, if this kind of inner conflict were allowed by nature, your body would quickly destroy itself in an internal war. Whatever thought system you are presently following may meet your needs today. However, tomorrow you might choose or be drawn to another level of consciousness—one more appropriate for new learning.

Ultimately, the spiritual path is actually a "journey without distance, to a place we never left." (*A Course in Miracles*) In other words, we *seem to be* on a path or journey, having experiences, learning lessons, and gaining knowledge. Yet, this path is merely part of the illusion of human perspectives and has no ultimate purpose. However, since we do *seem* to live in this illusion, the journey of spiritual evolution *is* necessary and essential because it is through this process that we create an opportunity to remember the Real World of God Consciousness. In so doing, all of humanity also attains this remembrance.

LEARNING: THE EASY WAY OR THE HARD WAY

While all paths eventually *do* lead to God, there are generally two roads or ways to travel the "spiritual path"—*the easy way or the hard way.* The easy way is to ask God to come into your life and for you to become a more conscious participant on your journey. In other words, it's about opening yourself to God Consciousness and letting It flow through all aspects of your being—physical, emotional, and intellectual. This path is made even easier if you have a greater acceptance, with little or no judgment, of yourself. On the other hand, the harder way is to evolve by trying to make all parts of yourself look better or reach a level of perfection. On this path, you are attempting to "spiritualize" the different parts of yourself. Yet, the truth is that even judging things as "unspiritual" is still a judgment.

I have known more men destroyed by the desire to have wife and child and to keep them in comfort than I have seen destroyed by drink and harlots. — **William Butler Yeats**

Whether you have chosen the easy way or the hard way, your goal has always been the same as that of students, disciples, initiates, masters, and ascended beings throughout time. It has always been about remembering who you really are and awakening that true Divine Self. As already stated, the fundamental difference between the two paths is that one is more painful *and* takes more time. Or it could be said that the easy way is to direct the light of the *heart downward*, while the hard way is *ground up* (pun intended). **When you grow tired of prolonging the journey or tired of the pain along the way, it's time to start making choices for the easier path.**

The theme of the easy path is that we are already whole and perfect beings with nothing to fix. In this state, we are not on a path of evolution, as there is already perfection. So, there is only one thing left to do, which is to let go and live according to what we believe is in alignment with being connected to God. However, since we seem to be in this temporal universe, the easy path encourages us to honor the illusion of evolution, while simultaneously living as though we were already connected. Yet, no matter how much importance we may place on the evolutionary process, we must never forget that it's all only a dream in the minds of God's children. Ultimately, learning lessons the easy way is like having a happy dream in contrast to the nightmare of learning lessons the hard way.

The easy path of spiritual growth can be summed up as *love and acceptance.* The most marked difference between the easy way and the hard way of spiritual evolution is that there is a lot less effort doing things the easy way. It means relaxing more and beginning to love and accept yourself, *as you are.* The easy way includes the choices that you make with the intention of expressing self-worth and love for yourself and others. The easy way produces and embraces miracles of transformation. This is not to say that you do not experience challenges. But when you hold more love and acceptance for yourself, even with your flaws, you have a far more enlightened perspective on what to change and how to go about it. Everyone eventually learns that **the path of** searching and unfoldment is really more about *remembering* a perfection once forgotten—not *finding* it. No one has ever discovered that the most efficient and effective path toward enlightenment involves obsessing over his or her flaws or being self-critical, as is done on the hard path. Instead, on the easy path, you realize that God is already present. Now, all that is left to do is open up and allow the Divine Presence to come through.

The hard path of spiritual growth, on the other hand, has two distinct stages. The first includes individuals who are spiritually asleep and not consciously participating in their evolutionary journey. They ignore or deny opportunities and callings for growth, thereby attracting harder lessons of evolution. The hard way basically involves choices that express fear, hate, and blame toward self or others, inducing karma and prolonging the journey of awakening. Those individuals who usually choose this more difficult path are often in denial or disinterested in their spiritual growth. Yet, even *they* will have their moments of awakening. Behold, the holy two-by-four awaits the christening to the head!

The second stage includes those who get "on the path" but tend to take it all a bit too seriously. This version of the hard way can be summed up as working hard to make yourself a "better person." All too often, these folks spend more time *working* on themselves or their lives and less time *enjoying* the lives they are supposedly improving. Once again, **the hard path consists either of the denial of the call for a spiritual awakening *or* the concealed belief that you must *earn* your way back to God.**

One example of working too hard on one's development is practicing abstinence in one form or another. This pattern of behavior includes individuals who think they must quit smoking or eating meat or having sex because they are now becoming too "spiritual" for all that. Then, of course, they not only try to abstain for themselves but they often try to convince others they should also do the same.

> *Who of you by worrying can add a single day to your life?*
> —Jesus (Matthew 6:27)

I once read about a study done on the value of working out. It was found that although exercise can lengthen your life span by a couple of years, you would have to spend the hourly equivalent of a couple of years working out. So, in the long run, you really only break even. The moral of the story is that if you have enjoyed working out, then you have *lengthened* your life and improved its quality, because you were having a good time while exercising. On the other hand, if you dreaded going to the gym (and eating all of those special green foods), then you actually *prolonged* your life and all its discomforts.

LIVING IN BALANCE

One of the most common realizations for students on the spiritual path is that living in balance is a vital key to discovering a life of wholeness. Living a life that is out of balance is a crisis waiting to happen. The severity of the impending crisis depends on how far out of balance you have become and for how long. Of course, the crisis is not always dramatic. Instead, it can sometimes be very subtle. Either way the crisis shows itself (subtle or dramatic), there is always time to change the course of things.

If you are, by nature, a more mentally focused person, then you will probably have less emphasis on some other aspect of your consciousness—such as your body. You need not condemn yourself if your body is not in great shape. You're simply seeing the results of being out of balance. If you want to change this imbalance, you need to shift your focus to include more physical activities. If you run every day, for example, you are naturally going to look physically better than someone who spends most of the day sitting behind a desk. You will never burn as many calories when you are reading as when you are jogging. Nevertheless, no matter which aspect of your being is getting the most attention, your focus will change when you want it to change badly enough. The primary goal is to live in balance.

If you don't like where you are in your life, then you need to shift the emphasis in your heart and soul (and allow a rebirth) rather than hold-ing your new life as a distant dream. Until that day of change comes, you must own the fact that you are allowing unpleasant experiences (which are really just symptoms of imbalance) into your life. This fact might be a harsh reality, but **if you want to know what is going on in your heart and soul, just look around you. If you don't like what you see, resenting it will not help—but *choosing differently* will.**

Ultimately, every soul on the planet wants balance, but most have forgotten how to find it. It is God's will that we all remember how to achieve this harmony. Once again, there are two ways to achieve bal-ance—the easy way and the hard way. When God works through you, God will encourage a balance of body, emotions, mind, and soul—earth, water, fire, and air. You'll spend time loving, forgiving, and learning to "empty your mind," for example. But you might also choose to include sex, exercising, inner healing, and journaling. Assuming that God will create this balance for you is not practical. As the saying goes, "Trust in Allah, but tie up your camel."

It might feel wonderful to say, "I just rely on God for my prosperity and abundance." But when the bank calls because you are overdrawn due to your not wanting to be "bothered" with such material things as balancing your checkbook, what will you do? Being too "airy fairy" is not living a balance of responsible spirituality; it's having too much air and not enough earth for grounding. Besides, if your spirituality is well *founded*, it should also be well *grounded*. Can you imagine trying to get the bank to neutralize your overdraft charges because you believe God is your accountant? It just doesn't work that way (although it might be fun to try)!

THE UNIVERSE IS A HOLOGRAM AND MIRROR

It's often said that the people and events around us are actually mir-rors for what is going on inside of us. This idea suggests the concept that the whole world is a three-dimensional hologram, projected from the souls of those who collectively perceive it. Or as William Blake ex-pressed, "We are led to believe a lie, when we see **with** and not **through** the eye." Even experiences within our own bodies and feelings (individually and collectively) are projected from inside our souls. When we look "out" into the world, we actually see things related to our own "inner" states of consciousness.

> *We do not see things as they are but rather as we are.*
> —The Talmud

Our experiences in the universe are a lot like watching films on a big screen. We are the ones who choose the movies being played. We are also the ones who write the scripts, direct the films, and even hire the actors. We dream up a false existence that we call the world or universe (which we mostly experience through our limited senses). Then we allow those senses to *interpret* our world. Finally, we learn to believe the feedback the senses offer us, which becomes the basis of what we call "reality." The soul, however, has higher senses that, when surrendered to God, reveal an entirely different reality or experience.

> *All we see or seem is but a dream within a dream.*
> —Edgar Allen Poe

Healing our lives and attaining mastery are about taking responsibility for our choices of dramas and actors. Since the outer world is nothing but holographic representations of our innermost thoughts and beliefs, our outer manifestations usually end up revealing inner parts of us with which we are least comfortable. However, these inner parts are mirrored in ways that we are most likely to learn from—whether we like it or not.

THE MANIFESTATION PROCESS

So, in the holographic mirror of human life, how does light become matter or, as the New Testament states, "the word becomes flesh"? (John 1:14) This law of manifestation is the same law that causes vibrations to become sound and love to express as service. As Edgar Cayce often emphasized, " . . . spirit is life, the mind is the builder [chooser]; the physical [manifestation] is the result." (349–4) Essentially, this statement means that **all of life's manifestations and experiences begin as pure Inspiration**. Then they either manifest *as* that purity (such as joy, love, and abundance) or take a turn for the worse (such as sorrow, hatred, and lack) at the level of the heart, or higher mind. If the latter choice is made, we allow ourselves to believe in the shadows of the world, rather than the Truth of Divine Origin.

It has been discovered in quantum physics that an observer's point of view determines what is seen. Therefore, if we change our thoughts and beliefs, what we manifest and experience will change. **When we stop identifying with the old and current concepts of who we are and surrender to the original (Divine) perspective, we become masters who radiate the light of God into the world.**

In the meantime, we experience *externally* (in the lower mind, emotions, body, and physical world) the life we create *internally* (in our hearts) and never by accident or coincidence. What we manifest in our material world is drawn to us because our souls believe that these experiences are what we need for our growth and the evolution of consciousness to the next level.

We are sick or poor or lonely because sickness or poverty or loneliness is serving the purpose of our soul.
—**Richard JoFolla**

2

Ancient Initiations

Every race and tribe, since the beginning of human evolution, has embraced some form of initiation into its culture. The term *initiation* simply means rituals of graduation—to some form of a higher level. In other words, we've always recognized that it feels as if we are missing something, *and* we want to remember *whatever* it is. Therefore, **spiritual initiations were, and always will be, about raising our spiritual level of awareness, with the ultimate goal of merging into the oneness of God.**

> *For you* grow *to heaven, you don't* go *to heaven.* —Edgar Cayce (reading 3409-1)

The sacred meaning of initiation has never changed. It was, and is, always about graduation to deeper and higher levels of awareness. The timeless value of initiations is shown in the parable, given by Jesus, of the king's marriage feast. This story tells of the great wedding where only those who are arrayed in the "golden wedding garment" can enter. On a symbolic level, this garment is prepared by consciously walking the spiritual path and integrating the lessons learned. Therefore, the parable tells us that to enter a state of heaven, we must pass through life's initiations and reach a level of spiritual attainment conducive to our goal.

ANCIENT CIVILIZATIONS AND ANCIENT INITIATIONS

It is believed by many that the first civilization on planet Earth existed in a land called Lemuria—a large landmass in the Pacific Ocean. This ancient culture is said to have existed from around 12 million B.C. until its final demise in 50,000 B.C.

The Lemurians were predominantly a very feminine, right-brain, and creative civilization. Yet, they were the first to develop initiations, which included sacred circles during solstices and equinoxes, at sites of sacred vortexes and grid lines on the planet. These ceremonies are still practiced by many groups today.

The Lemurian elders (mostly female) utilized toning, aroma, music, and vibration to enhance the effects of their gatherings. The primary goal was to evoke a spiritual awakening within the participants with the intention of activating a permanent shift in consciousness, toward a remembrance of their true, divine nature.

By the time Lemuria ceased to exist as a large continent and civilization, another culture known as the Atlanteans was well on its way to becoming earth's primary civilization.

The Atlanteans are said to have existed from around 200,000 B.C. to 10,000 B.C. on a large continent in the Atlantic Ocean, known of course as Atlantis. Once again, with the intent of evoking a heightening of awareness, the Atlanteans used initiations and ceremonies on a regular basis. However, being a more masculine civilization, the Atlanteans added more buildings, temples, and other structures to house their initiations.

According to Edgar Cayce, the Atlanteans had two primary temples of initiation. The first was known as *the Temple of Sacrifice*, which was used to cleanse and purify the dense body. The second was *the Temple of Beauty*, which was used to develop the inner self—emotionally and mentally. Later a Hall of Records was built in a location that would survive the eventual deluge (with the records of the Atlanteans and of humanity buried within it) in an area below the Sphinx, near the Great Pyramid of Giza.

When the Atlantean age came to a close around 10,000 B.C., there were numerous refugees who migrated to both sides of the Atlantic Ocean, bringing much of the Atlantean culture (philosophy, art, and technology) with them. This included the use of initiations and the high science of harnessing the celestial and terrestrial energies to enhance the potency of their initiations. Soon there were many new cultures spreading throughout the planet, taking the practices of initiation with them. As a result, Atlantean initiations can be traced into Greece, Egypt, Britain, Central and South America, North America, Africa, China, and throughout Europe.

The Atlantean rituals of development were so important that soon after arriving at new destinations, each of these surviving cultures built temples for their initiations. As was true for the Atlanteans, there was usually more than one temple, each with a different purpose or theme. Eventually the new cultures would alter some of the details of these initiations to fit the local region or blend in with the local customs, but the heart of the ritual remained the same. It was always about furthering the students' awareness of their true identity and role on the planet. Furthermore, the ritual always related to one of the four elements or four states of human consciousness.

The Native Americans, for example, developed the Sundance ceremony—as an earth-based ritual. The initiates of this ritual would have eagle claws attached to their breasts, with a cord attached to the tendon of the claws, and would be hoisted up into the air. As they were pulled up, the claws would grab in a little tighter. If the claws ripped through the skin, it wasn't time yet, and the initiate/student failed the test. On the other hand, if the student *was* ready for a vision, he would be hoisted up and spun around. After which, he would blow on a special ceremonial whistle to call in the gods and go into an altered state of consciousness. This is a spiritual ceremony, but a very physically oriented one.

In ancient Egypt, there were numerous temples of initiation. In fact, it is believed by many that the Nile River was symbolic of the human spine with temples actually built all along the river symbolizing the centers, or chakras, of the human energy system.

In some ways, we could say that individuals in the past were far more committed to their spiritual growth than we are today. **In modern times, most of the population practice some form of religion and/or spiritual ritual but rarely consciously apply the teachings in everyday life—which results in learning lessons the hard way.** They seem to lack the focus and commitment once seen as essential for true growth. In ancient times, on the other hand, when you went into a temple, you did so with full commitment. In fact, ancient initiations often involved life and death scenarios. So, it was clear that if you failed the initiation, you sometimes died. As you can imagine, this meant that only the few most *committed* individuals actually signed up for these types of spiritual initiations. It's one thing to go today and hear a lecture on emotional healing, but quite another thing, as in the days of the ancients, to enter a lion's den to see if you could process and clear your fear. Needless to say, in those days you had to be fully aware and very committed.

THE SACRED SYMBOLISM OF SOLOMON'S TEMPLE

For the ancient Israelites (and symbolically for all of humanity), one of the most revered temples of initiation was the sacred tabernacle, which became Solomon's Temple. It was in this temple that the Ark of the Covenant was housed. The sacred geometry of Solomon's Temple concealed numerous teachings, but only those with "opened eyes" could see and understand their significance.

According to some traditions, the layout of Solomon's Temple was as follows: The area surrounding the outermost walls symbolized the world outside and the unawakened portion of humanity. Next, the portion of humanity that was awakened, or at least on their spiritual path, was symbolized by those who were allowed to enter the main gate and participate in initiations. Within the main gate, there were, as might be expected, four initiations, which represented the four states of human consciousness, the four elements, and the four "beasts of Ezekiel." These four beasts are also the same as those of the "fixed" signs in astrology— bull (Taurus—earth), eagle (Scorpio—water), lion (Leo—fire), and man (Aquarius—air).

The first ritual, or initiation, involved the sacrifice of an animal, symbolizing the release of physical attachments. The second initiation involved a cleansing ritual in a large basin of water, symbolizing the healing and purifying of emotions. The third initiation involved the burning of incense to purify the mind. The fourth initiation involved a ritual with specially prepared bread that was raised only with air, symbolizing a purifying of the heart.

Ultimately, what the initiates of Solomon's Temple experienced was a symbolic journey into the root center (chakra) of the human body, where they began their initiations. Then they symbolically journeyed upward, through the navel center, the solar plexus, and finally to the heart center. There was, however, only *one* person, the High Priest, who was considered worthy of receiving the fifth initiation, which occurred in a room beyond a veil, or tabernacle curtain. This veiled chamber symbolized the Christ center (or throat chakra), as well as the three divine centers and initiations—collectively. In this room was the sacred Ark of the Covenant, which tradition says was used by the Israelites to commune with God.

Solomon's Temple was an external replica of the human body and its symbolic initiations. So, it is by no coincidence that within the human skull, there are seven primary bones joined together by a small winged-shaped bone known as the sphenoid. This bone, found behind the upper bridge of the nose, sits symbolically in the body's "holy of holies" (the combined three centers of Divinity) and has even been coined "the Ark of the Covenant" by some osteopaths and practitioners of cranial therapy.

Even the highly initiated master, the High Priest, was not considered to be *completely* prepared or worthy to enter the holy room. So he had to wear a special breastplate made of twelve uniquely cut and selected gemstones. This breastplate was, in modern terms, a lead shield to protect the wearer from radiation. Additionally, the High Priest had a cord bound around his waist. Then, if his own vibrations were not sufficient to handle the energy within the sacred chamber and his lead shield failed him, the assistants would drag his dead body out by the cord, since they were not allowed to enter this sacred room.

Symbolically, the inner chamber represents the head and neck of the body and its trinity of divine chakras, as well as representing heaven and the trinity of God. The veil that separated the assisting priests and all initiates from the sacred room symbolizes the veil that seems to separate us from Heaven. This is the same veil mentioned at the crucifixion of Jesus. As Jesus "gives up his ghost," the Bible states that the veil in the temple is torn open. This rending of the veil in the Holy of Holies symbolizes the present awakening and availability of Christ Consciousness and the worthiness of all people to walk into the remembrance of their Divinity.

SYMBOLISM OF THE CROSS AND SOLOMON'S TEMPLE

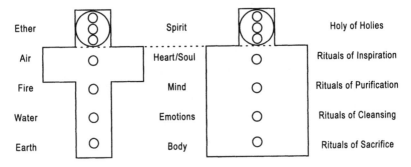

Ether		Spirit	Holy of Holies
Air		Heart/Soul	Rituals of Inspiration
Fire		Mind	Rituals of Purification
Water		Emotions	Rituals of Cleansing
Earth		Body	Rituals of Sacrifice

THE ESSENES

One of the last great ancient schools of initiation, prior to the time of Christ, was the Essene school and community of Qumran.

Until the twentieth century, little was known about this reclusive sect of masters. Scholars could only speculate their purpose and role in man's spiritual evolution. Edgar Cayce brought to light the metaphysical implications of the Essene existence. Cayce also accurately saw that women were members of the Essene community near where the *Dead Sea Scrolls* were discovered.

The Essene school began centuries before the time of Jesus. It was often referred to as the School of Prophets because one of its main achievements was to graduate teachers who often became biblical prophets. Among the last of such prophets was John the Baptist (as well as his parents), whom scholars now accept as being an Essene.

The primary purpose for the creation and existence of the Essene community was to prepare the way for the birthing and development of the one who would become the Christ. In fact, the name *Essene* means "expectant ones." Their role is confirmed by the fact that after existing for generations, they disbanded immediately after Jesus' crucifixion and resurrection as though their work was done.

There is much evidence that the parents (Joseph and Mary) of Jesus were also Essenes and that the Essene community was involved in their preparation to be the parents of the Christ. After enduring intense initiations, the day finally arrived when Mary was visited by an angel. The angel told her that, among several potential candidates, she had been chosen to mother the coming Messiah—the soul who would complete life's initiations and attain Christ Consciousness.

It is fulfilled.—Jesus (last words uttered at the Crucifixion—John 19:30)

The Holy Spirit also filled Mary, the mother of Jesus, because she was the highest initiate of all earthly women. She had most nearly perfected within herself the receptive, feminine aspect of the Christ Spirit. Mary was, by reason of this attainment, able to aid the Master Jesus in developing a body capable of holding and maintaining the Christ energy.

THE AWAKENING OF CHRIST CONSCIOUSNESS

A powerful shift (from outer to inner initiations) occurred 2,000 years ago with the initiations of Jesus. In His initiations, Jesus attained the level of consciousness referred to as "Christ Consciousness," meaning that He remembered His true identity. The events in the life of Christ outline the identical steps of other saviors *after* Jesus, but with this important difference: **Initiation is no longer** as dependent on outer rituals, or *external* **processes, as it is on** *internal* **experiences.**

Jesus is said to have completed his *inner* initiation into Christ Consciousness at the symbolic age of thirty-three, a number always held as the highest *external* initiation of the Freemasons and other esoteric groups. The number "thirty-three" secretly represents the symbolic evolution upward along the spine, which has thirty-three segments.

The early stages of the spiritual path usually take many years in comparison to the final stages. Note how Jesus' physical birth and water baptism were separated by thirty years, while the next steps were taken within three years. This difference in time demonstrates the concept that once you start to "get it," changes and awakenings begin to occur more rapidly.

The Aquarian Gospel of Jesus the Christ, by Levi H. Dowling, gives one version of the seven temple initiations that Jesus undertook. These are (1) Sincerity, (2) Justice, (3) Faith, (4) Courage, (5) Philanthropy, (6) Love Divine, and (7) Christ Consciousness. Every event described in the life of the Christ becomes an example of initiation within the body and life of each initiate. Now, we can all become a Christed one—a beloved child in whom our Divine Father is well pleased.

SINCE THE BIRTH OF CHRISTIANITY

Since the time of Jesus, the Christed One, there continue to be schools of initiation and great teachers who focus on Christ Consciousness. Some of these include the Rosicrucians, the Arthurian Knights, the Ascended Masters, the teachings of Ashtar, Edgar Cayce, Paramahansa Yogananda, and the teachings of Unity Church—to name a few. For those who seek other reliable sources of modern, Christ-centered material, there is no greater place to look than within. Whatever feels simple, clear, inspiring, and loving to *you* is probably resonating with your Christ-Self. **When something resonates with your Christ-Self, you are in the presence of the Christ.**

3

Modern Initiations

In some ways, it could truly be said that the initiates of old were far more committed to their spiritual paths. However, in other respects, today we are actually more evolved because we practice our initiations on a daily basis—albeit, not always consciously. **Each moment of every day, we are applying whatever level of spirituality we've integrated, whether we know it or not—even if the form may not look very evolved.** It's a lot like being asked to mathematically add something. We might still call on the crude system of adding on our fingers, while others can accomplish it in their heads. Either way, we will draw on whatever we have integrated as a tool.

Much the same, all of life's experiences are putting us to the test. We might be applying our spirituality on the freeways, at work, or in the schools. Yet, it's obvious we are now more advanced than the ancients. Rather than only a few individuals signing up for temple initiations as in times of old, our spirituality has become a part of our daily lives. Thus, humanity, as a whole, now participates in initiations more consciously and on a regular basis.

A NEW WAY

The old saying "the way to God is narrow" implied that enlightenment was only for a few but actually meant that only a few chose to listen. Now, we are *all* choosing to awaken—the easy way or the hard way. It's just a matter of time before our awakening reaches a point of "critical mass." Some people refer to this as the "hundredth monkey effect," wherein, when enough individuals wake up, the new consciousness is downloaded into the collective consciousness at a much faster rate—perhaps instantaneously. One of the greater implications here is that we are all in this together and are meant to wake up from the dream and return home. As the Bible states, "It is God's will that no soul shall perish." (II Peter 3:9)

The spiritual path of today takes many forms. In ancient times, you might go into a temple and deal with bottomless pits or be placed into a room with wild animals to learn about your inner fears. If you were fearful, you failed the test and could try again in the next lifetime. However, if you processed and quickly cleared your fears, you were doing well and survived. That's the way it was done in the old days—the original "school of hard knocks."

Today, when you lie down on a massage table or have someone work with you, saying: "Let's do some breathing here," you get in touch with this issue or that past experience or some emotional trauma. "Oh! Look! Some fear just came up. Okay, let's do some more deep breathing, apply some love and forgiveness, stay centered, let's move right through that." Now the fear starts to disperse, and you experience a transformation. You pay less than a hundred dollars, work on a fear issue, and feel pretty good about yourself. That's the way we do it today. Having created some *easier* ways, we are fortunate to have less life-threatening versions of spiritual evolution. Yet, even though today's initiations are seemingly less hazardous, they should not be taken for granted.

THE BODY IS A MAP FOR YOUR JOURNEY

In the initiations of the ancient past, we learned about our inner selves by experiencing rituals and ceremonies in the outer world. Now, it's time for everyone to realize that the treasure we seek is more easily found with a map. The map is hidden within your own being. When you are choosing to travel the road to self–improvement, like any other journey, it helps to use a map to understand where you've been, where you are going, and where you are—in relation to your destination. If you look at a road map, you might realize that your journey and the path you have chosen may have taken you through some rough terrain. But you can still reach your destination, even though for a moment you might have thought you were lost. **Similar to a road map, your body is a map with hidden esoteric symbolism that can give you greater clarity about your journey through life.**

The esoteric map (known as your body) can teach you about your life's direction. Of course, when you look at any map, nothing is seen as good or evil. It's merely about directions and destinations. Two of the most powerful keys to mastery involve knowing your destination and holding your focus on that goal. Then, once you create the focus or decide upon your goal, the means of attaining it becomes clearer. An understanding of this map can help you to identify the roads you have chosen, but perhaps without the judgments you may have had in the past.

When you are using a map, if you want to go north and see signs of traveling east, west, or south, you know it's not in alignment with your goal. It's that simple! There may be people and situations in your life that represent a direction you, as the traveler, can choose but are not in alignment with your higher goal or destination. **Travelers on the path of awakening must eventually learn to make choices that *assist* them in reaching their goals and also to choose *against* what-ever distracts them from those goals.** Ultimately, however, you are the one who makes the choice as to which road you take.

The body, when viewed as a map, reveals that the divine three centers (or chakras) of the head and neck symbolize your origin and ulti-mate destination. The four centers of the torso symbolize all the possible states of consciousness that you can experience as a human being and all the lessons involved with the spiritual evolutionary process. Furthermore, all of these paths relate to corresponding chakras (or energy centers) in the body.

An understanding of the body's esoteric symbolism is one of the most powerful keys to unlocking the mysteries of initiation. Symbolically speaking, when you are participating in ceremonies and practices that involve your body or the earth, you are entering a school that primarily focuses on your relationship to the earth/body. On the other hand, when you go into a school that stimulates your mind and/or how to use it to learn, heal, or manifest, you are in a school that mirrors the initiation of the mind. So, each path, religion, and philosophy has a theme.

If someone says, this school or that religion is better than another, you can see that one simply focuses on one particular subject or theme more than another. One is not better than the other. **Each school and path is spiritual. But they all represent one or more of the four states of human consciousness—physical, emotional, mental, and intuitive.** Buddhism, for example, is a very heart–centered thought system and focuses on compassion. Native American, Wicca, and Druidism, on the other hand, are very earthy and focus on ceremony and ritual. One represents an earth path, and the other is a heart path. They all represent areas equally necessary to becoming a whole, balanced being. You will be drawn to study the one you most need to learn. Just remember that, although you might place greater emphasis in one particular area at any given time, *all* the various states of your consciousness are always being developed to some degree or another.

An important key to unlocking the mysteries concealed behind initiations can be found in stories and mythologies. Some of the world's greatest teachers have used (and still use) parables, stories, and mythology to convey the deepest truths and awaken the listener. One such story or allegory is that of *Pinocchio*.

A MODERN PARABLE

1. Pinocchio's creator (Geppetto) gives him a body. Then, a spirit (a beautiful angel) breathes life into him. Soon afterward, he receives a conscience in the form of a little creature (Jiminy Cricket).

2. The creator (Geppetto) loves his creation but wants him to learn and therefore sends him to school.

3. Once Pinocchio departs, he begins to lose his focus and the purpose, or goal, given to him. Further, he often ignores his conscience that attempts to keep him on track. As most of us know, he soon finds that each time he is not truthful, his nose grows longer, which is symbolic of how the lies we learn to live will grow and grow until they can no longer be overlooked.

4. Eventually, Pinocchio falls to the carnival (or carnal-evil) and ends up at Pleasure Island. This leads to his being turned into a beast, or jackass (which is how we behave when we lose sight of our true nature). Yet, occasionally the messenger Jiminy Cricket (as Pinocchio's conscience) arrives to help him.

5. When Pinocchio finally escapes the imprisonment of Pleasure Island, he returns home to look for his father. But his father is no longer where he expects to find him. Now, Pinocchio must go within the sea of his unconscious self and through a life-and-death experience to find his creator.

6. Pinocchio and his father finally reunite in the depths of the sea. However, it's necessary to bring their reunion to the surface (or back home), a journey which symbolizes the need to integrate our spiritual awareness into our personal lives.

7. In the attempt to integrate his lessons, Pinocchio sacrifices himself—learning unconditional love. The angel brings him back to life because of his selflessness and makes him a real boy—an awakened being.

Pinocchio is one of the many stories and mythologies containing profound metaphors relevant to our own personal stories of initiation and unfoldment. These stories are designed to assist anyone who has the "eyes to see and the ears to hear."

4

The Variations of Human Consciousness

O ur progress on our spiritual journey is proportionate to our ability to understand ourselves and our various states of consciousness. According to esoteric traditions, we are made up of seven levels of awareness. Many thought–systems use the energy centers on the body (called chakras) to depict these seven states of consciousness. **The three upper centers symbolize the divine trinity of God *and* our three spiritual initiations. The four lower centers are symbolic of the four human states of consciousness *and* our four human initiations.**

The combined layout of these seven centers acts as a secret (sacred) key or map to our spiritual development. This map provides greater clarity in understanding how we evolve spiritually. It shows who we *really* are (our divine nature) and who we temporarily *seem* to be (our human nature).

Throughout this book (and in the art and science of sacred geometry), the circle represents God or God Consciousness. The dash line represents the veil between God Consciousness and the place of our human experience—the universe.

THE SYMBOL FOR GOD AND THE FIRST CREATION

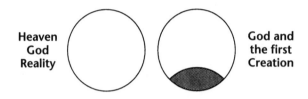

THE SEPARATION FROM GOD

We are and always will be in the presence of God. We are created within the heart and mind of God, and there we remain eternally. However, what *seems to be* is that we have journeyed away from God and Heaven. We are now seemingly on a spiritual path, search or evolution, with the goal of returning home. I emphasize *seems to be* because we are actually still in the mind and heart of God. But we've "made believe" we separated and are now evolving and earning our way back home—hence, the story of the Prodigal Son.

Further understanding of why this world, our bodies, and the universe are an illusion (only *seeming* to exist) and are often described as a dream or illusion is found in the book of Genesis. Here we read that before the separation of genders, and before the "fall" in Eden, Adam was put into a deep sleep. But nowhere in the scriptures does it say he woke up. This means that every object, emotion, and experience that ever existed since the creation of human consciousness has always been a part of the original dream.

Although we are and always will be in our Divine Spirit Consciousness made in God's perfect image, we seem to have passed through a veil of illusion. We are no longer in touch with our divine identity—our true nature. Instead we've taken on a new name or identity. Now, we see ourselves as merely "evolving" souls—trying to get back home. **Our four states of consciousness (body, emotions, mind, and soul) are symbols of where we seem to have gone since the moment of our original separation from Spirit.**

THE SYMBOL FOR TWO WORLDS: REALITY AND ILLUSION

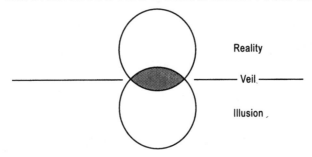

Despite any appearances to the contrary, to this day our connection to God is literally and figuratively as close as our connection to our bodies. The diagram below illustrates the line that represents or symbolizes the veil of illusion that seems to separate heaven (head and neck) from the world (the torso and its four centers of human consciousness). Again, the collective trinity (upper three spiritual centers) above represents the spiritual trinity of God and our divine self. The four centers below represent the four states of human consciousness. These combined, total the sacred number of seven and symbolize the seven sacred initiations.

The effects of this apparent separation are very similar to seeing pure, white light (our true self) beaming through a prism (the veil of illusion). The prism or veil causes the pure light to refract into numerous colors (states of consciousness). Although each color is made of the essence of pure light, no *one* color looks or feels like any other. This same process of one white light refracting into many colors holds true for us as well. The analogy of colors refers to levels of consciousness, not skin pigment. Rather than imagining each of us as represented by a different color of the rainbow, imagine instead that all the refracted colors sym-

MAJOR CHAKRAS WITH ELEMENTS ASSIGNED

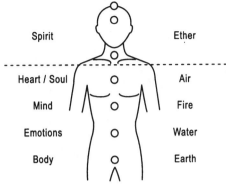

Spirit		Ether
Heart / Soul		Air
Mind		Fire
Emotions		Water
Body		Earth

bolize the various attributes (or states of consciousness) we all possess. When we see the world, we perceive it through the colored lens of our particular state of consciousness. So, what we see and experience depends on the clarity and color of our lenses. Furthermore, what we call life, the world, and our universe are holographic projections originating in our souls and projected through the lenses of our various states of consciousness. The world we see is through our individual lenses. The world we *all* see is through the combined perception and lenses of all souls.

PURE LIGHT THROUGH THE PRISM OF ILLUSION

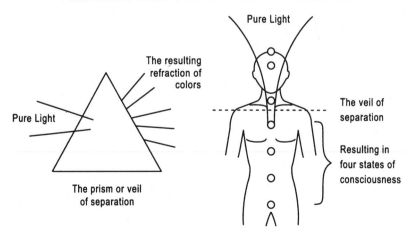

Pure Light

The resulting refraction of colors

Pure Light

The prism or veil of separation

Pure Light

The veil of separation

Resulting in four states of consciousness

THE SACRED SEVEN

In ancient times, the elders, teachers, and guides who facilitated conscious initiations knew intellectually, instinctively, and intuitively that the most sacred number for humanity was the number seven. This number has been revered above all others throughout history and occurs more frequently in sacred texts than any other. Therefore, it has always been the most consistently symbolic number for initiations. As Philo Judaeus of Alexandria wrote in the first century, "in Heaven, too, the ratio of the number seven begins and from there it descended to us also, coming down to visit the race of mortal men." Philo elaborated by saying that all beings divide into seven parts—internally and externally. Other ancient traditions held that there are seven sacred breaths, seven variations of voice, and even seven motions of the body. This sacred number is also seen in the seven–day story of creation, our seven days of the week, the seven major chakras of the body, and the golden menorah in Solomon's Temple, which had seven candlesticks. Also, there are seven primary notes in the musical scale, with the eighth note being the bridge to the next octave. Similar to the musical scale, the human cranium has seven major bones with an eighth bone connecting them.

Another example of the sacred number "seven" as it appears in the form of initiations is found in the Catholic tradition. There we find seven sacraments: *Baptism*—bestows grace at birth; *Confirmation*—gives the power of grace to adults; *Holy Eucharist*—integrates the flesh and blood of Christ; *Penance*—provides healing for the soul's wounds; *Extreme Unction*—gives the power for full restoration of the soul's health; *Holy Orders*—provides priests to teach, administer, and sanctify the mystical body of the Christ; and *Matrimony*—provides members for the new mystical body.

In more recent times, Madame Blavatsky (who formed the Theosophical Society) understood the sacred qualities of the number "seven" and related it to our esoteric and physical anatomy. Edgar Cayce explained the relationship among the seven chakras, the seven major glands of the body, and the seven churches of the Book of Revelation. A contemporary of Blavatsky and Cayce was Alice Bailey—one of the first clear and authentic channels of the Ascended Masters. Alice Bailey taught about the seven initiations of the human being (*Initiations: Human and Solar*). She said that the first initiation is related to overcoming the commands of the body, the second initiation is related to the subjugation of desires and emotions, the third initiation is related to the mind, and the fourth is related to the transfiguration of the soul. Bailey then grouped the final three initiations together and described them as a fine-tuning process.

THE MAJOR SPIRITUAL CENTERS

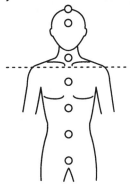

TWO TRINITIES DIVIDING ONE HEART

After our involution into matter, we found that we could no longer readily access our divinity. We could now, at best, only reach the heart center, which became the highest state of human consciousness. In our hearts, we found the new home for our "evolving" souls. Therefore, the heart center is traditionally accepted as the fourth, and highest, of the *human* chakras. Although our true nature is Divine Spirit, symbolized by the upper three centers in the head and neck, we now often limit our identities to mere human consciousness, symbolized by the four lower centers of the torso.

Of course, the heart can never truly replace our original divine self, but as many teachers and teachings often suggest, we can still search our hearts for a greater understanding about ourselves. The ancient Egyptians taught that the decision-making part of us is actually in the heart. This is because the heart is where our core beliefs are held; these beliefs result in the choices we make and the experiences we create.

Spirit is mirrored into the heart, then our decisions of the heart are mirrored downward into our human experience. When we allow Spirit to fill our hearts, the resulting manifestation in our mind, emotions, and physical world can be that of bliss and abundance.

In the heart center lies the superconscious self and what I believe *A Course in Miracles* refers to as the "home of the Holy Spirit." The ancients believed that the True Divine One never actually *incarnates* but only sends Its reflection downward—and does so into the heart. Some even taught that the Seven Aspects of the Elohim reflect into what they called the "seven brains of the heart."

> *The spirit moveth upon the heart, within the bosom of the heart.* — Jacob Boehme

Once we establish the heart as the new center and home of the soul, a new diagram becomes helpful. Our spiritual self (highest self) is still symbolized by the upper three centers, while the more human aspects of our identities and personalities (the intellectual mind, emotions, and body) are expressed and experienced through our lowest three centers (lower self). In between these two sets of centers (the upper three in the head and neck and the lower three within the torso) lies the heart. Here, in the heart, we find the soul—feeling torn between the two realms of heaven and earth, reality and illusion, divinity and human experience. The lower self (and its three aspects) mirrors the effects of what transpires in the heart. **Even though the heart center is merely one of the four centers of human consciousness, it is the home of our soul (higher self) and is now our bridge to reality.**

THE HEART AS OUR NEW CENTER

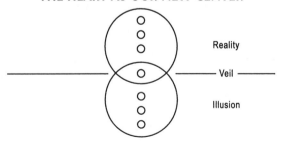

The viewpoint of seeing the heart as the home of the soul is expressed well in *The Upanishads* of the Far East: "The body is the city of Brahma, and in this city is the palace, the heart. So large is the space within the heart that both heaven and earth are contained within it, as is whatever there is of Him, and whatever shall be." This concept is very similar to the Taoist philosophy and the theories of Chinese medicine, which teach that Shen (Soul) is the ruler of the body and resides in the heart. Whenever there is peace in this ruler, there is peace in the whole kingdom.

When individuals make reference to their "higher self" (which could have several meanings), they usually hope to be referring to the deep recesses of the heart and soul—the *superconscious self.* Again, the higher self is found in the heart center. However, there are other levels of consciousness (besides the heart level) that are also "higher" than the material, conscious self—for example, the emotional *subconscious self.* Consequently, since even the emotional *subconscious self* is vibrationally higher than the physical, conscious self, some people might mistakenly refer to (and trust in) *any* voice other than their conscious mind as their "higher self." Fortunately, this too can be remedied by allowing God to be your Source.

THE SACRED FOUR

Once again, divinely speaking, you are Spirit, with a capital "S." You are perfect and whole and a part of God. The evolving you, the human you, however, is made up of four states of consciousness. These four states are the physical (material), the emotional (which includes the astral and psychic), the mental (intellectual mind), and the heart (intuitive or higher creative mind).

Philolaos, the Pythagorean (c. 400 B.C.), may have originally revealed the relationship between the four elements and the four states of human consciousness. He assigned the earth to the generative aspects of the soul, water to the passionate (emotional), fire to the intellectual, and air to the more spiritual. Some schools of thought eventually reversed the latter two, making the intellect or mind related to the highest element, air. However, this may have been merely an unsuccessful attempt to place the lower, intellectual mind in a higher status than the heart and soul.

In addition to their relationship with the four chakras and four elements, these four states of consciousness are also reflected in the sacred "four directions" of the Native American tradition, the four beasts of the prophet Ezekiel, and the four horsemen of the Book of Revelation. Therefore, the four elements (and other symbols of four) can also reveal information about your nature and spiritual journey. There is an earthly element to you, as well as water, fire, and air elements. The earthly state of consciousness represents the more physical aspects of life (such as the body, money, and sexuality) and correlates to the root center located at the base of the spine. The water element represents emotions and desires and relates to the navel center. Fire corresponds to the mind, willpower, and determination and is found in the solar plexus center. Air represents the more subtle and refined soul qualities of imagination and intuition, which correlate to the heart center.

There is a purpose for mastering each *one* of these four states of consciousness. However, like a wheel, each of these states also has many spokes or facets. For example, the physical state of consciousness (or root chakra) includes such facets as health, sexuality, money, and the will to live. You might become a master at one or any combination of these facets. The concept of spiritual evolution involves the mastering of several or all of the facets behind the primary state of consciousness to which they are related. Therefore, in the example just given, you would work to develop each aspect of the physical state of consciousness. So if you want to master the physical self, it stands to reason that you may also have to master its many facets as well.

THE FOUR STAGES OF HUMAN INITIATION

Physical Initiation (base chakra or state of human consciousness) involves nutrition, health, the will to live, money, vitality, sexuality, exercise, and getting in touch with your masculinity.

Emotional Initiation (navel chakra or state of human consciousness) involves emotions, romance, emotional healing, psychic development, inner child work, past traumas, and getting in touch with your femininity.

EACH CHAKRA HAS MANY FACETS

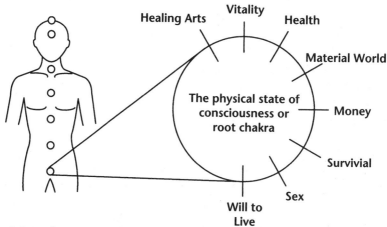

Mental Initiation (solar plexus chakra or state of human consciousness) involves willpower, positive attitude, study, intellectual development, reason, logic, focus, and organization.

Intuitive Initiation (heart chakra or state of human consciousness) involves developing humanitarian love, compassion, joy, unconditional love, creative arts, and care for plants/animals.

MY OWN EXPERIENCE OF THE FOUR HUMAN INITIATIONS

My physical initiations were primarily experienced in high school and the next few years thereafter. During this time, I studied and experienced martial arts, healing arts, yoga, and tantra. I also studied and lived the Essene way of life—which meant not eating meats and living closer to the earth. The healing arts I studied varied from herbology and massage to energy work and acupressure. This physical initiation lasted about five years. When it concluded (for the time being), I felt so healthy and energetic that I believed I was now a "whole and complete" being. It was also during this period of physical initiations that I began teaching health and healing-related classes, as well as martial arts.

The emotional and psychic initiations I experienced overlapped slightly with that of the physical—especially since I was studying psychology and parapsychology, while also learning healing arts. This new initiation began when I entered a bookstore to buy yet another herbology book. I overheard a discussion between the clerk and a customer, who was describing a metaphysical university where she taught classes in psychic development. I was intrigued enough to approach her and register, right on the spot, to be her student. This class began my studies that would culminate in a degree in metaphysics near the time I finished college.

While attending the school of metaphysics, I learned every imaginable form of psychic reading/divination—from cards and astrology to I Ching and bumps on the head (phrenology). I also learned numerology, smoke readings, tea leaf readings, face reading, and much more. At this point, I was certain that now I must be a "whole and complete" being. So, I set out to open a school wherein I could teach more extensively.

Although the transition from the physical to the emotional initiation was exciting and fairly smooth, such would not be the case for *any* of the initiations that were still to come.

The initiation of the mind, as I experienced it, was the result of an unexpected turn of events that would result in my having the good fortune of being introduced to one of the great spiritual *minds* of our time—Manly P. Hall. He would become one of the many masters of the mental initiation who helped to define this aspect of my consciousness.

The door of my mental initiation was now wide open. I studied philosophy, the works of Joseph Campbell, sacred geometry, Science of Mind, secret societies, and numerous related topics. My personal library soon grew to thousands of books, as I did all I could to absorb every form of spiritual teachings available. I also developed the use of the mind for greater focus and for "creating the life I wanted."

Ahhhh! Now, with my body and physical self all in order, my emotional awareness and psychic skills developed, and my knowledge and the powers of my mind intact, I was finally a "complete and whole" being. Or so I thought.

After spending years in the mental initiation and becoming a seasoned speaker, teacher, and healer, the hardest initiation of all (for me) was about to take place—the heart initiation.

The initiation of the heart (and soul) is unlike anything else you can experience because it awakens creativity, unconditional love, and a sense of oneness with all of life. However, this initiation also triggers an experience often referred to as "the dark night of the soul"—which is how it happened for me. The "dark night" aspect of the heart initiation usually takes the form of having your life fall apart in most or all areas, which can make you really question all that you had previously learned. The most well-known accounts of such an experience are that of Job (recorded in the Bible) and St. John of the Cross, who wrote *The Dark Night of the Soul.*

What is to give light must endure burning. —Victor Frankl

Such difficult periods of our lives are often misinterpreted as resulting from God's wrath or judgment for our sins. But nothing could be further from the truth. We are the ones who call forth or attract these lessons because we believe they will teach us something we need to learn.

Ultimately, the purpose for this period of cleansing (through the heart initiation) is to learn: (1) to be less attached, (2) to be more unconditional in our love and sharing, (3) to integrate all that we have learned and experienced up to this point in our lives, and (4) to prepare us for the three spiritual initiations that represent our awakening into Divine Awareness.

Part III

The Four Human Initiations

This section explores the four primary initiations or states of human consciousness. Each of these initiations relates to one or more of our spiritual centers (chakras), which have always served as part of our esoteric anatomy, acting as a map for our spiritual journey.

The four chapters in this section (Chapters 5–8) give a more specific account of each of the four human initiations and their respective spiritual centers. Each of these chapters begins with an introduction and explains what the reader might expect to encounter during these initiations. Then, the chapter closes by revealing some of the perks and pitfalls of working on the particular level of consciousness discussed within the chapter. Relevant gemstones and music are also noted that could enhance the evolution of any particular level of growth.

It cannot be stressed enough that the teachings and teachers recommended in this book are only a small sample of possibilities. The list itself could have filled a book. Therefore, it is crucial that you discern what kinds of teachers and materials feel right for you and which states of consciousness they might represent.

It also needs to be clarified that although this book presents the spiritual centers and respective initiations in a chronological order (that is, from the anatomically lowest to the highest), your own life's initiations will probably not occur in this same order. Instead, your initiations will come to you in the order that your soul sees necessary for your highest good. Further, it is common for individuals to work within one initiation, seem to move on to another, and then find themselves back at the first to develop greater clarity and understanding. Lastly, although in the near and distant past, individuals would choose (or be selected for) a specific level of initiation, today it is far more common for people to experience more than one level of initiation at a time.

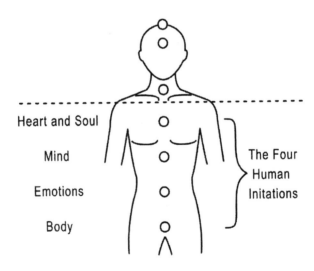

5

First Initiation: The Body–Earth

The initiations and developmental stages of the root chakra and our physical state of consciousness are represented by our physical world and physical bodies (as well as the etheric body). **The moments of your life that represent initiations of a physical nature are quite varied but similar in that they all have to do with your body and/or the physical world.** This initiation can be experienced and expressed as sex, physical workouts, health consciousness, special dieting, and earth rituals, as well as struggling with illness or practicing healing arts.

The body (and the physical world) can accurately be referred to as an illusion and should, therefore, never be given priority over a spiritual focus. Our bodies (and the world) are just shadows in the dreams of our souls, shadows that we allowed to control us. Yet, without first healing our misperceptions of the body and the world, the greatest heights of spiritual awareness cannot be reached. Therefore, the personal transformation we are all seeking is very much dependent on the transformation of our bodies. This transformation process is enhanced by love and acceptance, which means learning to love, nurture, and embrace the body, the world, and all their attributes. Also, the body and the world around us are perfect external mirrors to show us how we are doing internally. In this sense, the physical world is valuable but only as a messenger. Yet, it is the message that holds the treasure.

Although some spiritual experiences are far beyond the limits and understanding of the physical plane, many of them must still be brought to earth, grounded, and channeled into something practical and applicable. In fact, the greatest masters are not necessarily the ones who detach *from* the world and their bodies, but instead are those who manifest their spirituality *into* their bodies. In so doing, they bring spirit to the temporary world of form.

HOW IT LOOKS

For me, the physical initiation began when I was in high school (and the first few years thereafter). At this time, I studied numerous healing arts, yoga, tantric sex, martial arts, herbology, and the Essene way of nutrition. I loved that part of my being—my physicality—and devoted most of the hours of the day to these studies. I found the most excellent books, teachers, and schools available. I wanted a good foundation, so I chose to work with masters in whatever field I studied. This lifestyle externally symbolized and manifested my inner process of a physical initiation.

With great enthusiasm, I set out to understand and master my body and the physical world. I had my "trusty" case of herbs, studied martial arts, and explored my sexuality. After several years, I had experienced many aspects of physicality. Eventually, there was a delusional period of time when I believed that if I learned just one more healing art or developed just one more aspect of my physical being, I would then be an absolutely *perfect* person. It was only a matter of time before I discovered that there were other states of consciousness to experience—beyond the body.

GETTING IN TOUCH WITH YOUR BODY

Sometimes, when working on your physicality, you may be drawn to the healing arts, either by studying them or receiving them. In other words, if your *body* is involved in an experience, then your soul is trying to learn about the physical body or about the material world. It's as if you are saying to the world and yourself, "I want to understand who and what I am—physically." Of course, there's an easy way and a hard way to learn. The easy way might be to go to school or open a book and study the human body, sexuality, prosperity and money, or anything else physical or material. However, there's also a hard way. This difficult path pays a visit to people who are receiving, but ignoring, the message to learn more about accepting their physical self and end up at the doctor's office or in the hospital to do so.

In essence your soul is saying, I must understand myself "physically" to get to know myself "spiritually." So, you're either going to hear the call and open up to the process or you're going to go "kicking and screaming" with resistance. Either way, there is a lesson that you need to learn. You may have heard someone say, "The universe told me to take a break, but I didn't. I guess now, with this broken leg, I am *really* getting a break." The bottom line is that your soul is aware of a needed lesson, and it will send this impulse into your life. The more you deny or resist, consciously or unconsciously, the more drastic the form of the lesson.

> *Your body may still create its own illness in response to a belief system. Compassion does not judge the illness. Rather, the illness is viewed as a response to a given belief, a pointer to know of the validity of the belief and its healing.* —Gregg **Braden**

You are not a victim, and the universe is not taking advantage of you. **There is a purpose to everything you are experiencing. Your soul calls forth experiences it believes will create the most effective and efficient opportunities for learning.** Whether you are someone who is studying a healing art or you are a heroin addict, you are *still* a person who is initiating—physically. The person in either example is seen by God as wanting to understand him- or herself and is using the body as a means to do so. However, one is choosing a more painful route than the other, but neither is judged as good or bad. **Know that everything you have done and experienced in your life can, and will, eventually be used for a higher good.**

Getting in touch with your body can also symbolize getting in touch with your physical/masculine nature. In one of the "lost gospels," Jesus tells the apostles to make Mary Magdalene into a man. He was referring to helping her to get in touch with her latent second half—the masculine aspects of her consciousness. Awakening both the feminine and masculine aspects of our inner self includes blending the creative right side of the brain with the logical left side. This balancing of the two gender polarities was also recommended by Jesus to the male apostles who needed to integrate more of their feminine, receptive natures. Jesus was implying that to receive higher teachings, we must all access a greater sense of wholeness.

GETTING GROUNDED

The physical initiation has two primary facets. The first is the physical body, and the second is the material world at large. In other words, for us to attain a healthy balance of our physical state of consciousness, we must first balance these two facets. Although the first initiation is the most fundamental, it usually proves very challenging. The hidden reason for this difficulty lies in the esoteric symbolism of the root chakra and all that it represents (such as money, sex, health, fitness, etc.).

The root chakra sits, anatomically, at the farthest possible distance from the divine centers. This placement leads to an unconscious judgment of the root center and all that it represents as being bad, lesser, unclean, and even shameful. Yet, it is an essential part of our awakening to release this stereotype, reclaim the root facet of our lives, and allow our spiritual presence to descend into our bodies and the material world. This is what it means to "get grounded." Once the root chakra is awakened and brought into healthy balance, our bodies and world quicken to a whole new level of presence and abundance.

The purpose of the material world is to get more material. — Swami Beyondananda *(New Age Comedian)*

THE LIMITATIONS OF THE BODY

The body has more limitations than any other aspect of human consciousness because of the density of its vibration. Some mystics have described the material world as "frozen thought." Of itself, the body is not alive, nor does it truly create. It only follows the conscious and unconscious demands of the higher human aspects. The body and the physical world have no real power. They (like the emotions and lower mind) are only holographic images that reflect our beliefs, thoughts, and feelings.

The same holds true for concepts of sex and money. Neither the physical aspect of sex nor the material possession of money should be seen as an end in itself. Rather, each one is a means—merely another wonderful tool or symbol with which to lovingly communicate and share our presence in the world.

Those who see with eyes of understanding, the difference between the body and the spirit within the body, and understand the process of liberation from the bondage of the material nature, attain the supreme goal. — Bhagavad-Gita

As mentioned earlier, just as some people neglect their bodies, there is also the opposite extreme: those individuals or groups who make the body their greatest priority. **Excessive focus on the body is just as out of balance as the other extreme of neglecting it.** Attaining mastery is about balance. To obsess on your diet, calling this food good and another bad, brings you *out* of harmony. It's far better to be a loving meat–eater than a judgmental vegetarian. In other words, you will *never* reach spiritual enlightenment by "perfecting" the body! Worrying about perfecting the body to extend your life is counterproductive and, in fact, is destructive. Instead, you can choose to be more accepting of yourself and others. Acceptance brings greater health and vitality to the body, while worrying, on the other hand, breaks the body down. So let go of trying to control the body and its fate. After all, if you're meant to be shot, you'll never drown!

If a pill does any good, take it, but gradually try to lead the thought from where it is into the higher realms of consciousness where the soul recognizes its own I-Am-ness. — Ernest Holmes

THE GIFTS OF THE BODY

Some people, consciously or unconsciously, assume that if they choose the spiritual path, they should spend their time either reading or meditating, and they therefore neglect their bodies. However, the body is equally important; it is one-fourth of our human consciousness wherein we live and manifest our spiritual experience. Besides, it is never by coincidence or accident that people allow the neglect of their physical selves. It often happens because it's a convenient way to escape some issues or opinions they harbor about the physical realm of life. These inner issues could be guilt, shame, or even low self-worth and could be connected to such outer issues as sex, finances, or physical appearance.

In cultivating the mind, we must not neglect the body. Those who do not find time for exercise will have to find time for illness. — John Lubbock

However, when issues such as these are brought to a reasonable level of healthiness and when Spirit is allowed to express itself through the physical level of our consciousness, the body and the material world are transformed into glorious experiences. In this state, there is a sense of purpose, good health and vitality, financial affluence, joyful sensuality, and a brighter environment.

When kept in balance and treated as a vehicle for expressing love in the world (for ourselves and others), the body, together with the physical world, can serve as a symbol of love and wonderment.

MODERN PARALLELS

In the Holy Grail legends, the physical initiation begins first when the knights make the mistake of confusing the symbol of the Grail (Christ) with a physical object. Then the knights mount their horses (another symbol of the material, animal-self) and venture off into their physical initiations. They are confronted with death and disease, and most of them die without ever finding the object of their quest. Hence they fail their tests—temporarily.

In the movie *The Wizard of Oz*, Dorothy chooses to leave "home"—resulting in a long quest to return. The physical aspects of her quest are demonstrated by her bodily illness or fever (which we learn about at the end of the story) and the *death* of the Wicked Witch of the North. It should also be noted that Dorothy (like many characters in popular mythologies) has an animal companion. In her case it's not the horses of the Grail knights, but instead a little dog that is as frail, yet inquisitive, as is Dorothy. Also, on her journey she is given a pair of beautiful *red* shoes to wear—the color usually attributed to the root chakra.

In *The NeverEnding Story*, a little boy is feeling small and inadequate, and other boys are picking on him. So he hides from the abuse by reading fantasy stories, which creates an escape or dissociation from the body. In one such story, he finds another version of himself as Atreyu, a young warrior and strong hero. Atreyu is ready to take on the quest of saving Fantasia, the realm of human imagination, which is on the verge of destruction. Ironically, the very thing that is destroying Fantasia is called "The Nothing," which, however, is probably the most accurate name possible for the evils of the world.

FACETS OF THE BODY—EARTH

The initiations of the first state of human consciousness can include lessons or studies related to the body, the earth, or anything of the material world. To enhance your awareness of this physical facet of yourself, consider reading books related to the body, the earth, healing, sexuality, and prosperity. You might also explore studies or practices such as dance or movement, martial arts, earth religions, fitness, health.

The facets noted as representing this center and initiation are only examples and are not complete. They can easily be added to and subtracted from, as per your own experience and perception.

Other methods of enhancing your physical self include: colors—red and earth-tones; music—rock-'n'-roll or rhythmic; instruments—drums; gemstones—bloodstone, garnet, and obsidian.

FACETS OF THE ROOT CHAKRA

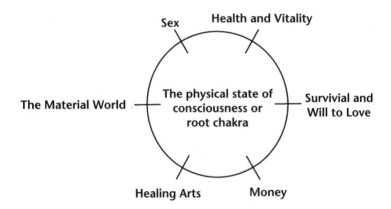

6

Second Initiation:
The Emotions—Water

The initiations and developmental stages of the navel chakra and our emotional states of consciousness show up in two different forms. **The navel center (found in the lower abdomen) manifests in two ways because it symbolizes both our emotional *and* psychic selves.** Of course, psychic gifts can accurately be connected to any and all of the other chakras and glands of the body (for example, pituitary or thyroid glands), but it's the navel center that primarily *symbolizes* the psychic state of consciousness. The navel chakra is the center of the psyche (pronounced *psych-e*), which includes things of a psych–ological or a psych–ic nature and their related arts and fields of study. Of course, most psychologists would not appreciate being categorized with psychics, but they do have similar roots of study: the sensitive, emotional facet of the soul.

When the second initiation manifests as *emotional learning and process-*

ing, it can take the form of working with relationships, rebirthing, counseling, inner-child work, or hypnotherapy. This initiation is also about getting in touch with one's true emotional and feminine nature, a work which includes greater sensitivity, emotional honesty, and vulnerability. The tests of the navel center are passed only after you have learned some level of emotional responsibility.

On the other hand, if the second initiation accesses more of the *psychic side* of emotional growth, your exploration might take the form of psychic development: channeling, past-life investigation, or any other tool of the psyche or the subconscious self. At this point, you might be going to psychic readers or learning how to do readings yourself. This psychic aspect of personal growth, like the emotional, is strongly connected to what is commonly referred to as *the subconscious*.

HOW IT LOOKS

The emotional stage of my own initiations involved the study of psychology and the preparation to become a counselor. Yet, all of the time I spent learning to heal others emotionally with counseling skills and developing my *psychic* abilities conveniently allowed me to avoid working on or fine-tuning *my own* emotional self.

Feelings buried alive never die. — Karol Truman

Sadly, I would discover that most psychics, spiritual teachers, and healers make this same mistake of not doing more *personal* emotional work. The confrontation with my emotional self could not be avoided forever, however, as I was eventually thrust into a deep healing process.

When I studied the psychic arts, once again (as with my physical initiation) I jumped right in. After enrolling in a metaphysical school, I studied every imaginable form of psychic development. The schools I entered taught everything from astrology and card readings to face readings and psychometry. It was an incredible experience and taught me how to use numerous tools to access the psyche of myself or others.

It was time to gain a greater understanding of the part of me that is beyond the physical, conscious self, for we are also subconscious (emotional, astral, and psychic) beings. So I believed that if I could just get this psychic and emotional state of consciousness all cleared and understood, then I'd be a complete and total being—still not realizing that there were other states of consciousness waiting to be explored.

THE DIFFERENCE BETWEEN EMOTIONS AND FEELINGS

Most people erroneously equate emotions with feelings and use the terms interchangeably. While they are similar in some respects (both are about "feeling"), there are distinct differences as well. It could be said that the feelings of the heart are a more intense version of those in the emotional center and are far deeper and more authentic. Eckhart Tolle, in his book *The Power of Now*, describes it as follows: "Love, joy, and peace . . . are not what I would call emotions. They lie beyond the emotions, on a much deeper level . . . The word [emotion] comes from the Latin 'emovere,' meaning 'to disturb.'"

Some of the feelings of the heart are so deeply hidden within the soul, they may go unnoticed. For this reason the soul will eventually need to bring them down into the emotional center and closer to the world of manifestation in order to make them perceptible to our conscious self. Emotions of the navel center and feelings of the heart center also have vastly different effects on the body and well-being. For example, because our emotional center is much closer to the physical center, emotions have a more direct and distinct effect on the body, while the feelings of the heart can be far more subtle (but not altogether unnoticeable) in their influence.

The emotional center is found in the lower abdominal region and is related to our more limited, emotional behaviors and reactions. Emotions from this center are mostly acting as a *mirror* of our soul's experiences—being either that of connectedness (love) or separation (fear). Feelings of the heart, on the other hand, are more directly related to the core of the soul and can express a sense of joy and connectedness that the emotional center could never comprehend. As Eckhart Tolle writes, "Love, joy, and peace are deep states of Being or rather three aspects of the state of inner connectedness with Being."

A good example of this distinction between the two centers is evident in how the unconditional love of the heart center will digress into a more conditional, restricted expression of love at the emotional level. Although both centers can express love, one does so in a higher, purer form.

> *When you look at things emotionally, you will not see them clearly; when you perceive things spiritually, you will understand.* — Peace Pilgrim

THERE ARE ONLY TWO EMOTIONS

Some say that there are only two emotions: love and fear. In truth, there is only one emotion with two facets. That one emotion is *love*. The first facet of love is where love is experienced. The second facet of love is the *cry for love* (when it is perceived as absent). God created love, but humanity created the second facet—fear. Both facets are *still* love—one, where love is present, and the other, where it seems absent. In addition to the emotional level, love and fear are also found at the level of feeling (in the heart), but as "feelings," they are far more intense (or deep) than the emotions found in the navel center.

> *God did not create in us the spirit of fear; but instead created power, love, and a sound mind.* — The Bible (II Timothy 1:7)

Although there are really only two emotions (love and fear), these two emotions breed a whole host of others, from the sublime and/or positive (passion, happiness, and feelings experienced when singing, dancing, and listening to music) to the primal and/or negative (lust, anger, loneliness, and hatred). But these emotions are *still* only depicting our soul-level choices to be connected (love) or separated (fear).

The seeming absence of love, or God, causes people to become afraid. When people are afraid, they become hurt and then angry, which results in numerous forms of hostile behavior. But it's still all rooted in the mistaken assumption that God and love are missing.

To overcome fear, so fill the mental forces with that of the creative nature as to cast out fear; for he, or she, that is without fear is free indeed, and perfect love casteth out fear.
—Edgar Cayce (reading 5439-1)

Poetry and music are two excellent examples of modes for expressing both oneness and connection or separation and loneliness. Either of these can be experienced as healthy or unhealthy emotions. Some poems and songs express a healthy feeling of connectedness. Others are clearly an unhealthy cry of longing for something outside of oneself. In the end, both expressions are beautiful if seen in the proper light. One speaks of love, and the other is a cry for love. The first is healthy, and the second sends a message that can also result in healthiness but only if the cry is answered appropriately—by reconnecting to the Divine.

THE EMOTIONS BEHIND RELATIONSHIPS

Because of our attachment to the archetypal fantasy of how relationships *should* look, the emotions behind personal relationships might be the most difficult topic to review. However, it is agreed by many healers and counselors that the most widespread addiction on the planet is codependency—which is an emotional dis-ease that stems from a sense of inadequacy or a belief that you are missing something *and* that someone else can fill that void for you. This inner discomfort manifests as the common quest for a partner, romance, and a much-needed reminder that you are lovable and desirable. Therefore, most relationships are more often about *feeding* this addiction and not about *sharing* sincere, mature, and authentic love.

The very thing that gives you pleasure today will give you pain tomorrow, or it will leave you, so its absence will give you pain. And what is often referred to as love may be pleasurable and exciting for a while, but it is an addictive clinging, an extremely needy condition that can turn into its opposite at the flick of a switch. —Eckhart Tolle

This is not to say that emotions are not valuable. Indeed, when the emotional center of consciousness is allowed to reflect an *authentic* level of spiritual love (as originally experienced in the heart), then this heart energy is channeled into the emotional center, manifesting as love-based passion and sensuality. Then your friends and lovers are not *needed* and viewed as objects from which you "get" something, but rather are chosen as someone with whom you value and *share* each experience. Said another way, **emotions (like the mind and body) are most healthy and harmonious when they dance to the music of the spirit and soul. Otherwise, when cut off from the True Self, emotions express as a constant struggle with addictive behaviors that result in depression and loneliness.** For this reason, the vital center in the navel region is also called the "hara," which is known in Oriental healing arts (as well as martial arts) as the center of gravity or balance. When we are not centered properly, emotionally and psychically, then we are off balance and vulnerable to attack, trauma, and sickness.

THE LIMITATIONS OF EMOTION

The emotional aspect of human consciousness is nearly as much an "effect" of our thinking or state of being as are the body and the material world. Although some people place great value on emotions and believe they can be experienced independently of our minds and bodies, emotions (like the physical body) are actually an effect, more than a creative force. Our bodies and emotions are like sensors for the soul and are two of the primary ways that we relate to our environment. Nevertheless, neither the body nor emotions exist independently from the soul. The soul, on the other hand, is independent and lives on beyond the life spans of our bodies and emotions.

> *Our feelings were given to us to excite to action, and when they end in themselves, they are cherished to no good purpose.*
> —**Daniel Sanford**

There are two kinds of emotions that create the greatest limitations in our lives—aggressive emotions and passive emotions. *Aggressive emotions* show up as hate and violence, as well as strongly addictive desires, and often take the form of victimizing others. *Passive emotions* are those mostly related to the hurts and resentments we hold inside. These ofttimes hidden emotions continue to affect our lives and make us feel stuck in negative patterns and scenarios that usually lead to living the life of a passive "victim."

What we typically refer to as love is usually a limited version of a far deeper experience and rarely reaches the level of Love Divine, which is all-inclusive and unconditional. This *limited* version of love is offered to some people in various measures and not at all to others. The love of the heart center, however, is far closer to Love Divine than the distinctly human love of the emotional center. Human, conditional love is a very limited perception of love's true potential, which can only be experienced when it is expressed unconditionally—*from* the Spirit and *through* the heart.

The Greek demigod Phaeton—son of the sun—convinced his father to allow him to drive the sun's chariot across the sky. He lost control of the horses, causing the sun to come too close to the earth and burn it. The horses in this story are a great analogy for losing the grip on our spiritual focus (from a lack of emotional maturity), resulting in our being controlled by emotions rather than having them serve us.

> *. . . influences in the emotions, unless they be governed by an ideal [spiritual focus], often may become as a stumbling-stone.* —Edgar Cayce (reading 1599-1)

THE GIFTS OF EMOTION

When we think of the gifts of emotion, it takes only a moment to see that they usually evoke concepts of human love. We might recall moments of being appreciated or being excited at hearing some good news or perhaps the feelings of a new romance. Some people even believe we can never understand Divine Love without first knowing the human emotion of love. However, this is not the case.

We do not learn about (unconditional) Divine Love by experiencing (limited) romantic, human love. In fact, the opposite is true. The human expression of love is only a *reflection* (and not a cause) of our inner development and experience. Human love doesn't *give* us anything that isn't already there. And since we already have all that we need, the ultimate fusion of love that occurs between two people does so when the expression of human love is *surrendered* to Love Divine. Then, a new level of understanding and experience takes place, raising the level of awareness within each person, which is then brought back into the human expression because of a permanent shift within. This view, of course, does not fit the model of romantics who feel as though they have a greater degree of love *because of* what some event or person has given to them. Instead, Love Divine comes from releasing the notion that there *is* any *one* or any *thing* else outside of us.

Some people also believe that one of the greatest gifts of emotion is *in* the emotional experience itself. In other words, just having emotion, be it joyous or painful, is a sign of "being alive." They might argue that even "the dark night of the soul" (which helps to open the heart) would not be possible without such emotions as despair, sorrow, regret, and unfulfilled longing. However, once again, emotions have a limited purpose and should be seen as merely indicators of our *inner* experience and not as having the power to control us or dictate our responses. Yet once we *do* experience negative emotions, a purpose can be made for them, which is that of being danger signals or wake-up calls. So, the *limitations* of emotions are most prevalent when we give them power over us, but the *gifts* of emotions are experienced most when we recognize their role as signposts or our soul's barometer of connectedness.

Another way to understand and appreciate the potential gifts of emotions is to realize that emotions can mirror our healthy decisions in life—not just our unhealthy ones. **When emotions reflect our heart-level decisions to know and experience who we *really* are, they can magnify the inner joy (of our hearts) into emotional passion and the thrill of being alive.** This internal change descends into our physical being and literally bathes our DNA and the cells of our bodies with love and life-force. Here is where the true value of *feeling* comes to light. This exhilarating renewal vividly portrays how it is that the choices we make (in our hearts and minds) have a tangible effect on us (emotionally and physically).

So, emotions *are* an accurate mirror of our choices and beliefs. They reflect back what we are holding in our hearts and the kinds of experiences we are creating in our lives. Emotions are like valuable nerve endings that warn us of a hot stove and show up most significantly to alert us when we are experiencing a lack of love and safety. But these same nerve endings allow us to feel the warmth of the sun as it shines on our skin after feeling physically cold (or emotionally frozen).

MODERN PARALLELS

In the Holy Grail legends, the initiation of emotions is portrayed by the Grail knight Percival, who is young and naïve. He is thought to be gullible and inexperienced with life. In fact, some mythologists believe that Percival was immature and had not yet experienced a rite of passage (initiation) to wean him from his mother, which temporarily prevented him from passing this initiation. She was thought to be *emotionally* overbearing and overprotective in an effort to keep Percival from meeting the same fate as his father, who died as a knight.

In *The Wizard of Oz*, the emotional initiation is depicted in Dorothy's moments of sorrow and longing for home. She manifests a cowardly lion that symbolizes a part of her that lacks emotional courage. Dorothy continues to push through her feelings but is still plagued by doubts and fears throughout the story. This is a great reminder that although we might pass a test on some levels, it can, and often does, repeat itself for us to get the lesson at deeper levels.

In *The NeverEnding Story*, the initiation of emotions is portrayed during Atreyu's dramatic experience in the "Swamps of Sadness." He loses his horse (symbolic of letting go of one level of initiation to enter another), as it sinks into the swamp with Atreyu crying, "Don't let the sadness of the swamps get to you." This is a message for us all. It encourages us to be aware of deep emotional issues that, when left unhealed, can rise over our heads and drown us.

FACETS OF THE EMOTIONS—WATER

The initiations of the second state of human consciousness can include lessons or studies related to emotions or psychic development. To enhance your awareness of this emotional facet of yourself, consider reading books related to codependence, the inner child, channeling, E.S.P., and reincarnation. You might also explore studies or practices such as hypnotherapy, counseling, healing trauma, rebirthing, astral projection, and dream interpretation.

The facets noted as representing this center and initiation are only examples and are not complete. They can easily be added to and subtracted from, as per your own experience and perception.

Other methods of enhancing your emotional or psychic self include: colors—orange and florals; music—romantic, blues, and country western; instruments—guitar and keyboards; gemstones—carnelian, coral, moonstone, cats-eye, and pearl.

FACETS OF THE NAVEL CHAKRA

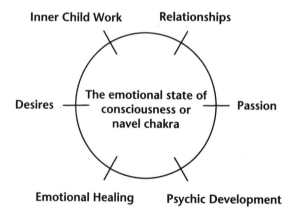

Inner Child Work   Relationships

Desires   The emotional state of consciousness or navel chakra   Passion

Emotional Healing   Psychic Development

7

Third Initiation:
The Mind-Fire

The initiations and developmental stages of the solar plexus chakra and our mental state of consciousness are most commonly related to the intellectual self, sometimes called the "lower-mind," in contrast to the "higher mind" of the heart center. While it's true that this solar plexus chakra/center is also often seen as an emotional center, it still symbolizes the mind. In fact, some ancient teachings refer to this center as the "abdominal brain" because it represents our intellectual and thinking functions.

The term *solar plexus* means center of fire or the fire element. The solar plexus is a complex network of nerve fibers of the sympathetic nervous system. It is composed of material similar to that of the brain. Also, like the brain, the solar plexus center both receives and transmits nerve impulses. Yet, this center of the lower mind is also, paradoxically, often associated with emotions—especially fear. The mental center being related to the emotion of fear may sound like a contradiction, but it actually makes sense because in our greatest times of fear we typically go into a thinking mode to try to escape (by flight) the feeling of danger. This is because the solar plexus is anatomically related to our adrenals, which are our "fight or flight" glands. The fears that cause this natural response in the body's endocrine system are attempting to be resolved by the primal, lower-mind, because when we are afraid, we often use *thinking* as a coping mechanism. In other words, when we experience fear, the feeling manifests in the solar plexus because we are trying to incorporate the lower mind's assistance in handling the emotional discomfort. However, even though the solar plexus region is related to our emotional fear response, it does not establish this region as the primary center for *all other emotions,* such as sadness, happiness, or loneliness. These other emotions, of course, would be found in the second (emotional, navel) center.

Initiations of the mental center are also commonly experienced during times of studying or reading. Buying lots of books when you already own several books that remain unread is a symptom of going through the mental initiation. Development of the mental state of consciousness is also evident when you notice you are placing a greater emphasis on the "power of the mind." This aspect of **the mental initiation includes self-empowerment training or most self-mastery seminars and thought systems.**

> *The more power one gives to his thought—the more completely he believes that his thought has power—the more power it will have.* —**Ernest Holmes**

Another vital aspect of the mental phase of growth is the development of focus and willpower. In fact, the skill of focus is probably the most important tool for all students on the path, going through any initiation. The ability to focus is what divides students from masters. As the Jedi master Yoda proclaimed, "Do, or do not. There is no try."

> *Abraham Lincoln's principle for greatness can be adopted by nearly everyone. This was his rule: Whatsoever he had to do at*

all, he put his whole mind into it and held it there until it was all done. — Russell Conwell

The Grail knight Percival's initial failure to attain the Holy Grail resulted in part from a lack of focus. He was not able to reach the necessary level of focus and mastery because he still had some unhealed emotional issues and weaknesses. Then, when he attained more mental focus and strength through healing, he passed his tests.

Unless one conceives of himself as possessing good things, he will not possess them. — Ernest Holmes

Other symptoms or aspects of experiencing the initiation of the mind include the development of organizational skills, linear thinking, and attention to details, as well as reason and logic. The initiation of the mind might also include such studies as Science of Mind, sacred geometry, and metaphysical sciences (like astrology and numerology).

This level of initiation clearly involves studies that are more intellectually oriented. It doesn't matter what the focus of your research is—be it God or science. A scientist is definitely mind oriented, but so is a positive thinker who uses the "science of affirmation." One peers into a microscope to discover the answers to one's questions, while the other searches religion or philosophy for answers to these same questions. Whatever form this searching takes, it's all still about the soul using and developing the mind as the vehicle for learning.

HOW IT LOOKS

When I entered the initiation of the mind, I began an intense period of reading and studying that covered a wide range of subjects, from ancient civilizations to sacred geometry, and philosophies to world religions. This phase coincided with my progression from a part-time to full-time spiritual teacher.

The third initiation was very appealing to my mind and certainly had a profound effect on me as a teacher. Also during this time, I encountered some amazing people who were masters of the mental level, including Joseph Campbell and Manly P. Hall. These masters had, as you might imagine, vast knowledge, focus, and a "bird's-eye view" of life. However, while the mental initiation intrigued my mind, it did not fill my heart; and this eventually led to yet another initiation—that of the heart.

TRIAL BY FIRE

For both men *and* women, the initiation of the mind is primarily about awakening traits of knowledge, focus, and determination. The ancients often depicted this mental level of development and awakening of personal power as a trial by fire. The Bible and "lost books" of the Bible tell stories of men being cast into a fiery furnace but not being consumed—an obvious portrayal of a fire initiation. Elijah's ascent into heaven in a chariot of fire describes another fire initiation. Both of these examples depict the heroes of the stories achieving success over their tests or transcendence over their trials through a spiritual illumination—nurtured by *focus and determination.*

HOW THOUGHTS MANIFEST AS THINGS

Another necessary part of developing the mind and passing mental initiations involves the understanding and proper use of the mind as a tool. **Thoughts create and attract mental molecules, which are charged according to the vibration of our mental impressions.** After the mental molecules are charged, they begin to attract other molecules of the more dense emotional and physical realms. Therefore, a positive thought creates a healthy physical manifestation, and a negative thought attracts an unhealthy manifestation. The stronger the thought, the more powerful the results. It also helps to keep charging the thought molecules (through repeated focus) to keep their effects from fading.

> *I visualized where I wanted to be, what kind of player I wanted to become. I knew exactly where I wanted to go, and I focused on getting there.* — **Michael Jordan**

Additionally, our thoughts collectively charge the molecules in the area around us. The more positive our thoughts, the more positive our life and environment. This positive atmosphere also has a very uplifting effect on the people around us, as they can choose to absorb these vibrations. In fact, if the skill of creating positive thought forms is adequately developed, we can literally direct our thoughts of love and healing toward others, which they can receive depending on their consciousness and receptivity.

When we are thinking negatively, on the other hand, an energy field of these thoughts surrounds us and tends to hover about until our guard is down or we are off-center. At this time, the surrounding negative energy backs up on us and invades our consciousness. Then, old habits or patterns can return from "out of the blue," or perhaps we might create or attract a trauma or crisis. Whatever the outcome, the apparent negative form could only arrive at our door if we have first sent out a message for it.

THE LIMITATIONS OF THE MIND

To say that the mind has limitations may sound like blasphemy to teachers and students of mind-power skills who claim to have harnessed the *unlimited* power of the mind. However, even the mind has potential pitfalls. The mind, like any other human expression of consciousness, can be ruled either by Spirit or by the ego. **There is a point where the mind has to be trained to focus and take action, and a time when it needs to be left quiet to receive new insights and inspirations from God and from the heart.** As *A Course in Miracles* states, "The miracle comes quietly into the mind that stops for an instant and is still." Yes, the mind *is* truly unlimited, but *only* when we surrender it to be filled with the unlimited power of God, Divine Guidance, and Inspiration. This is appropriate humility.

> *It has been said that we can know God only insofar as we can become God . . . It is to be taken figuratively and not too literally, for we cannot really become God, but we can and do partake of the Divine Nature.* —**Ernest Holmes**

As many students of spirituality and self-help programs have discovered, if left unchecked, the lower mind makes itself a *god*. It can become an inflated, controlling, and fearful voice whose advice is limited to primal survival functions—never at peace and always anticipating its next threat. In fact, the lower level of the mind is closely related to the primal, fear-based, reptilian portion of the brain. This is why *A Course in Miracles* refers to the lower mind as the ego's home or domain. However, the functions of the lower mind can be evolved or raised. When this occurs, all the mental development once used for personal grandiosity is turned around and surrendered to a higher good.

Another pitfall of becoming overly attached to the power of the mind is the common tendency of becoming too mind-dependent, while neglecting the physical and emotional self. For example, if suddenly you are gaining weight or getting sick more often, it might mean that you need to pay more attention to your physical self. Perhaps you have forgotten about living in balance because you are focusing so much attention on reading or positive thinking. No matter how much success you have had with developing your mind, it is still important to nurture equally *all* facets of your life and being.

THE GIFTS OF THE MIND

As previously stated, one of the most important gifts of the mind lies in the ability to use it to focus one's thoughts, feelings, and actions. As Pascal once stated, "Man's greatness lies in his power of thought." The mind can be used as a disciplinarian to slow down or eliminate the erratic energies of the world to make room for God. Some refer to this process as focusing the manic mind. Then, in the resulting silence, we can experience inspiration.

> *It's all right to have butterflies in your stomach. Just get them to fly in formation.* —Dr. Rob Gilbert

Another gift of the mind is its ability to choose. This important function is well illustrated in the story of Alice in Wonderland, wherein Alice asks the Cheshire Cat which road she should take. He responds by telling her that it all depends on where she wants to go. When she replies that she does not know, he tells her that it doesn't really matter which road she takes then. The lesson here is that we have to learn to make decisions *and* take responsibility for the choices we *have* already made. If we truly want to awaken from the dream of pain, limitation, and separation, we must make the choice to do so.

MODERN PARALLELS

In the Holy Grail legends, the initiation of the mind is illustrated best as the Grail knight Percival begins to develop a more mature sense of focus and courage. He demonstrates his growing awareness and moral strength when he uses his willpower to refuse the distractions of the maidens he encounters, as well as the temptation to betray his king. He also uses his developing mental power to keep focused on his quest for the Grail.

In *The Wizard of Oz*, Dorothy experiences the initiation of the mind when she attracts a companion who is looking for a brain. The scarecrow, who lacks a brain, represents a part of her she finds incomplete. This story reminds us that it is possible to experience messages and lessons vicariously through other people or even objects outside of us. Initiations need not always occur directly within our own bodies or minds, but instead are often mirrored in the people and world around us.

In *The NeverEnding Story*, the mental level of initiation is demonstrated when the hero, Atreyu, must get past a pair of giant statues that come to life when they sense someone passing who does not recognize his or her own self-worth. If the initiate *fails* the test, the sphinxes shoot fire (symbolizing the third chakra of mind) from their eyes, burning anyone who lacks focus and finds him- or herself unworthy.

FACETS OF THE MIND—FIRE

The initiations of the third state of human consciousness can include lessons or studies related to developing the mind. To enhance your awareness of this mental facet of yourself, consider reading books related to willpower, sacred geometry, lost civilizations, quantum physics, and metaphysical sciences. You might also explore studies or practices such as self-empowerment, goal setting, personal mastery, and religious science.

The facets noted as representing this center and initiation are only examples and are not complete. They can easily be added to and subtracted from, as per your own experience and perception.

Other methods of enhancing the mental aspect of your soul include: colors—yellow and bright shades of many colors; music—jazz and progressive rock; instruments—horns; gemstones—opal, amber, fire agate, and citrine.

FACETS OF THE SOLAR PLEXUS CHAKRA

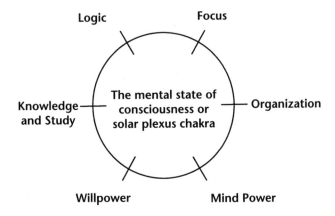

8

Fourth Initiation:
The Heart and Soul–Air

The initiations and developmental stages of the heart chakra, and our intuitive and creative state of consciousness, are the final of the *human* initiations. This heart level opens us up to our higher mind, but not as yet our divine mind. **It is from our hearts that we ultimately make our life–decisions because this center is the symbolic home of the soul.** So here we make our decisions to be guided either by God above (located in the trinity of the centers in the head and neck) or by our lower self (the mind, emotions, and body). The latter case is warned about in the Bible: "The fool has decided in his heart, there is no God." (Psalms 14:1)

Signs of going through a heart–level initiation "the easy way" could involve experiencing a period of newly developed or heightened creativity. Another sign is motherhood (or fatherhood) which, for most women (and some men), awakens the heart center to a much deeper level. Other possible signs and symptoms of opening the heart include events or studies that awaken compassion, unconditional love, forgiveness, and surrender. **The mind learns by studying, but the heart learns by integrated experience.**

> *The best and most beautiful things in the world cannot be seen or even touched. They must be felt with the heart.*
> —Helen Keller

As the result of heart illumination, Gautama Buddha declared that his teachings, called the "Noble Truths," were not derived from any "handed–down doctrine" of the mind, but that "there arose within him the eye to perceive them." Compare the Buddha's statement with what the mystic Jacob Boehme said of himself, "I am not collecting my knowledge from letters and books, but I have it within my own Self; because heaven and earth with all their inhabitants, and moreover God himself, is in man."

> *I received most of my knowledge from God, rather than from books . . . I tell you what I have perceived directly. That is why I speak with authority, the authority of my direct perception of Truth.* — Paramahansa Yogananda

What about doing heart–level initiations the hard way? Since in the heart–centered initiation you cannot learn unconditional love with all of your past opinions clouding your understanding, what often happens is that many of the people and things you are most attached to are inevitably taken away. This forces you to learn one of the primary lessons of the soul—to let go of *attachments.*

The heart–level initiation is sometimes referred to as the initiation of Buddha, since it involves the development of compassion, humanitarianism, and a sense of oneness with all life. However, the difficult aspects of this initiation are also reflected in some of the challenging tests that Gautama Buddha endured, including the separation from his family when he embarked on his spiritual path.

The lessons and initiations of the heart center mostly involve the purging away of the lower self through learning the futility of being driven by its impulses. Needless to say, this purging (which is like a purification) can manifest in the loss of many or all of the things to which the lower self is attached. These lessons can seem very painful but can teach us to learn how to call upon a higher interpretation of whatever we are experiencing.

Blessed are the pure in heart, for they shall see God.
—The Bible (Matthew 5:8)

HOW IT LOOKS

For me, the heart initiation was the most difficult of all. I experienced this level by its traditional name, "dark night of the soul." As the Bible's Book of Psalms reflects: "Yea, though I walk through the valley of the shadow of death, I will fear no evil, for Thou art with me." (Psalm 23:4) My "dark night" involved numerous losses and hard times, which ultimately taught me to let go of attachments *and* identification with my lower self.

During these difficult times, I found that the books I enjoyed during the mental initiation were of little assistance. They could not rescue me from the depths of pain and frustration that are a part of this initiation. Fortunately, however, I found one exception—*A Course in Miracles*—which opened my heart to new levels of understanding, as well as methods of applying love and forgiveness. As the saying goes, "The truth will set you free, but first it will *really* piss you off." **The heart and soul initiation encourages us to let go of teachers and books (although only temporarily) and, instead, become the *embodiment* of what we read or learn.**

My own personal initiation of the heart and soul can be summed up with a dream I had during this period. In the dream, I entered a temple where masters approached me. With my left hand, I presented my certificates of achievement as statements of my (first chakra) experience, since I assumed that this is what they wanted to see. After all, the world usually judges us by our appearances and experiences.

Man looks at the outer appearance but the Lord looks into the heart. — The Bible (I Samuel 16:7)

Consequently, the masters in the dream refused my offering. Then, I extended my right hand, which was filled with all of the psychic tools (second chakra) I had collected, including my tarot cards and psychology questionnaires. Once again, my offering was refused.

So I thought I would really impress them by presenting a huge stack of books, representing the many hundreds I had read and knowledge (third chakra) I had acquired. Yet, again, the masters of the temple would not accept my offering, which was necessary for my admittance into this temple.

Seeing my despair and confusion, the masters said, "This is a temple of the heart. What do you know about matters of the heart, such as love?" When I realized that they were not asking me about tantra (first chakra), nor about doing a reading (second chakra) on the love in a relationship, nor the definition as found in one of the books I had read (third chakra), it occurred to me that I had no answer. So the masters patiently showed me a simple act of love and reached out to share a hug. However, I realized that I could not hug them while my arms were filled with all of my accumulated certificates, tools, and books. Then, one master spoke up saying, "It is also true that you can never really experience love while you are still filled with the objects and experiences of the past."

The lesson here is that it is necessary to empty the old contents of your cup before God can refill it with new understanding. As Joanna Rodgers Macy wrote, "The heart that breaks open can contain the whole universe." You have to put aside the things previously learned and experienced when you want to discover what love truly is (and we all do). Otherwise, **you will inevitably revert to former experiences to define love until you learn a new version.** So when the initiation of the heart calls you to learn about love, you may, at first, automatically offer your past references of love—defined sexually, emotionally, or even intellectually. But eventually, you'll learn a new heart-centered version of love—commonly referred to as unconditional love. This new level of true love is whole, sensual, serving, and inviting. It fills the pages of mystical poets like Rumi. John Lennon also captured it well in the song "Across the Universe."

A dream or vision is all fine and wonderful, but what was happening in my waking life was not so great. Like the man named Job of the Old Testament, I was purged to the bone. I was feeling a sense of hopelessness. I was also feeling anger, grief, and guilt for having spent so much money and time on books and schools, learning things that were not helping me with this dark experience. I felt defeated until I had a vision wherein God told me that I had not failed but that I had to stop trying to impose perfection on an imperfect world. It was a message about learning the true meaning of *acceptance*—another key lesson of the heart.

> *When your illusions clash with reality, when your falsehoods clash with the truth, then you have suffering.*
> —Anthony DeMello

Eventually, I realized that one of the primary messages of my heart initiation was to "let go and surrender." It was a time of learning to let go of my own accomplishments and to trust a Higher Power. It was time to do less *for* God and more *with* God.

> *I know God will not give me anything I can't handle. I just wish that He didn't trust me so much.* —Mother Teresa

THE DARK NIGHT OF THE SOUL

The initiation of the heart is similar to being crucified, and it feels that way too. As the saying goes, "Religion is for people who fear hell, but spirituality is for those who have been there!" It is, to be sure, a time of death—a death (or transition) of the old self—which makes room for the new self to be born. True rebirth actually occurs in the *initiation of Spirit* that is to follow (hence the term "spiritual rebirth"). However, in the initiation of the heart, the way is *cleared* for this transformation.

> *Doubt along the way will come and go and go and come again*
> *. . . When you forget, remember that you walk with Him and*

with His Word upon your heart. — A Course in Miracles

During this period, you are experiencing a test in surrender and un-conditional love, which means letting go of the tools and coping skills you formerly relied upon. So the car or body breaks down, the house goes, the marriage falls apart, and your emotions and relationships go haywire. Then the mind goes next. All that you thought you knew in-tellectually doesn't work to heal matters of the heart center; or as Pascal once said, "The heart has its reasons, reason knows not of." Remember that you will always be learning, but you have a choice to learn the easy way or the hard way.

During the dark night of the soul, you will feel like a major part of you is dying—and it is. But it's a part that you truly want to let die, or let go of—even though you might not always realize this consciously. We further complicate things by clinging to that which is trying to die. Of course we do so because we are afraid of letting go of our familiar past. Jesus vividly described it when he said, "He who wishes to save his [old] life will lose it." (Luke 9:24) So you feel the pain that only comes from a lack of surrender or from clinging to your old patterns. However, remember that since this world of illusion *is* (by its very nature) only temporary, so are all of the threatening circumstances that you might encounter. In other words, "This too shall pass."

It's within your heart and soul that you choose to either be the per-fect and complete being God created or rely upon the "new," separate self who searches the world to fill a lack that was/is never really there. You either stay aligned with God's version of who you are and learn the easy way or you re-create yourself and learn the hard way. Remember, you are always learning, but you can choose to "go with the flow" of Spirit or resist it. Although these trials and tribulations of the dark night of the soul may sound discouraging, there is a powerful message be-hind them. This message is about letting go of a fear-based life and old perceptions. It's about surrendering to a Higher Power that may have seemed far away or even nonexistent but is drawn closer by the very act of surrender. So do what you can to be at peace during these troubled times, because they occur for a reason.

Blessed are those who mourn, for they shall be comforted.
                                   — The Bible (Matthew 5:4)

YOU ARE UNIQUE

No one in the world has had exactly the same experiences you have had. Your own experiences make up a part of the unique person you are. At any moment, you can choose to shift your life from painful and nightmarish experiences to the "happy dream" version of who you are. Then, inevitably, you can say, "I've gone through a lot of challenges and my life has been really tough. But I got through it!"

> *Hail to you, gods, on that day of the great reckoning. Behold me! I have come to you, without sin, without guilt, without evil, without a witness against me, without one whom I have wronged.* — The Book of the Dead

Keep in mind that there are many people on earth who are still in a struggle similar to what you have gone through. They could benefit from someone saying, "You know what? There is another way." They might not listen to someone else who hasn't had the experiences *you* have had. So, you see, we all have a soul's purpose. Ultimately, it is to bring the Light and Love of God into our lives and into the world. This is the *collective* soul's purpose, shared by us all. However, your *individual* soul's purpose is to manifest that love in your own unique way. Furthermore, because each of us has had unique experiences, we all have something special to bring to the world and in a form and style that no one else can. Pretty empowering, isn't it? So **there is always a soul (or group of souls) out there who needs exactly what you have to offer.**

MYSTERIES OF THE HEART

Humanity has become so mind dependent that it's almost terrifying to some to conceive of letting the heart become the more accepted guide. After all, the mind is known to be a problem solver, which is what we think we need when we are in crises. Consequently, we have learned to rely on logic rather than wisdom. The art of letting go and letting God illuminate our hearts with the all-knowing wisdom of the ages has become a rare thing indeed.

> *The way of Heaven can be known and experienced through the heart.* — Manly P. Hall

The heart teaches forgiveness, compassion, creativity, trust, and imagination; but humanity is rarely taught the usefulness of such traits in matters of daily living. Nevertheless, there is a mysterious power in trusting the wisdom of the heart. The masters of ancient times (including Moses and Pythagoras) were often called *magi*, which referred to their profound level of wisdom and initiation. They used their hearts as their guide rather than the lower mind. The term *magi* is also the root of our word *i-magi-nation*. **Imagination is one of the primary aspects of the heart chakra and heart initiation.** It is one of the most overlooked and powerful tools available to us—which prompted Albert Einstein to say, "Problems cannot be solved by the same minds that created them." In fact, Einstein's theories often resulted from imagination and visualization. To better understand his theories of traveling at the speed of light, for example, he asked himself, "What would it be like to be riding on the end of a light beam?"

The new wave of children being born today have chosen to more freely express their heightened state of imagination. This same choice is also available to people of *all* ages and cultures. We have evolved to a point where we can more easily commune directly with God and connect with the nature of our own hearts.

> *I will put my law in their inward parts, and write it in their hearts, and I will be their God and they shall be my people.*
> — The Bible (Hebrews 8:10)

So mysterious is the heart center that an ancient secret society (known as the Rosicrucians) taught that within the heart exists a "seed atom." The seed atom is like a spiritual flight recorder that holds all of the data of your soul's many journeys, adding to the wisdom and sense of inner knowing often attributed to the heart. When you die physically, the flight recorder, or seed atom, is withdrawn through the "silver cord," which is said to connect your soul to your body. This process has commonly been referred to as "your life flashing before your eyes." After this life review, the silver cord is severed, and your soul departs from the body, along with its personal files. The information in these files is a part of your soul's ongoing memory and eventually becomes a part of the collective memory of all souls throughout time. These compiled records are known as the Akashic Records or the Book of Life.

THE LIMITATIONS OF THE HEART

Few students or teachers on the spiritual path would dare to say that the heart has its limits. Nevertheless, it's true! The first limit of the heart worth mentioning is that, although the heart contains ancient wisdom and a record of *all* human experience, the heart is *still* only as old as the created universe. Only when it is open and surrendered to the Divine, does the heart access wisdom beyond time and a "peace that surpasses understanding."

Another limit of the heart is that this center of consciousness has all too often become the hiding place for those who would deny the other, seemingly lower aspects of human consciousness—such as the body. If a person truly has some level of avoidance of the physical or emotional aspects of consciousness, rest assured there is a reason—possibly some form of physical or emotional trauma or abuse, either past or present.

> *People always say, "Let your heart tell you what to do." Well,*
> *your heart sometimes is bruised and it doesn't serve you well.*
> **—Kevin Costner**

An imbalance or avoidance of the body and emotions can take the form of a person being extremely creative but out of touch with more practical life issues (such as finances)—hence the term "starving artist." At some point, such people decided that the world was not a safe place, except within their own dissociated citadel in the clouds. This reaction to the traumas of life is completely understandable. However, the healing and wholeness of any person are greatly dependent on the ability to bravely reintegrate into the world, where a better life awaits.

THE GIFTS OF THE HEART

The gifts of awakening the heart center are beyond measure. As Charles Dickens wrote, "A loving heart is the truest wisdom." The opening of the heart center is synonymous with the quickening of the soul. It is not something that can be faked or contrived, nor is it fleeting or temporary. The love of an opened heart center is real, authentic, and powerful.

> *Though I can speak with the tongues of men and of angels, and have not love in my heart, I am merely sounding brass or a tinkling cymbal. And, though I have the gift of prophecy, and understand all mysteries and knowledge; and though I have faith enough to move mountains, I am nothing. And though I bestow all my goods to feed the poor . . . and have not love in my heart, I gain nothing. Love is long-suffering and kind; love does not envy . . . is not easily provoked, thinks no evil . . . but rejoices in truth . . . Love never fails; but whether there be prophecies, they shall fail . . . whether there be knowledge, it shall vanish away . . . And now abide faith, hope, and love . . . but the greatest of these is love.*
> —The Bible (I Corinthians 13:1-6, 8, 13)

MODERN PARALLELS

In the Holy Grail legends, the heart initiation is portrayed by the Grail knight Percival, who is young and naïve, lacking groundedness, and showing signs of being too "airy fairy." As stated earlier, he is thought to be gullible and inexperienced with life. Yet, despite having symptoms of an imbalance in his heart center, Percival is known for being innocent. Some legends refer to him as the "guileless fool," or as having an innocence commonly referred to as "pure in heart."

In *The Wizard of Oz*, Dorothy encounters yet another projection of herself and her own lessons in the form of the tin man who is looking for a heart. It should be noted that the tin man feels empty and is literally hollow without a heart.

In *The NeverEnding Story*, the initiation of the heart occurs when Atreyu has a vision of himself in a frozen mirror. This scene is symbolic of the need to be willing to look within our hearts and souls to discover our true natures and deepest fears. As Carl Jung said, "Your vision will become clear only when you can look into your own heart."

FACETS OF THE HEART AND SOUL—AIR

The initiations of the fourth state of human consciousness can include lessons or studies related to the body, the earth, or anything of the material world. To enhance your awareness of this imaginative facet of yourself, consider reading books related to creativity, visualization, angels, compassion, and forgiveness. You might also explore studies or practices such as Buddhism, *A Course in Miracles*, creative arts, Taoism, and journaling.

The facets noted as representing this center and initiation are only examples and are not complete. They can easily be added to and subtracted from, as per your own experience and perception.

Other methods of enhancing the heart aspect of your soul include: colors—green, pink or salmon, and pastel shades; music—classical and new age; instruments—strings; gemstones—emerald, malachite, watermelon tourmaline, rose quartz, and jade.

FACETS OF THE HEART CHAKRA

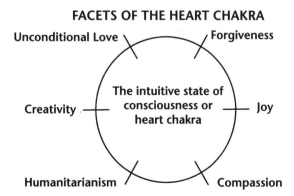

Part IV

The Three Spiritual Initiations

This section explores the last three (of the seven) initiations of spiritual growth. While the first four are initiations of human consciousness, these three represent the trinity of spiritual initiations. As a reminder, although there *seems* to be three spiritual initiations, there is really, in many respects, only *one*. Just as the four human initiations are closely related, so too are these three, but to an even greater degree.

The first of these three spiritual initiations is that of Christ Consciousness (Chapter 9), wherein students are introduced to their Divine Self—the part made "in God's own image." (Genesis 1:26)

The second initiation of the spiritual trinity focuses on integration (Chapter 10). The lesson here is that no matter how much you experience a spiritual awakening and no matter what level of "mastery" you might achieve, it all has to be *integrated* as a permanent part of your being. **All initiations, no matter how simple or how profound,**

must be *integrated* into your life and become a part of *who you are*. Lessons that are not integrated are "filed away," as lessons *still* needing to be learned. The integration referred to in the fourth initiation (Chapter 8) differs from that in this chapter because the former refers to integration of your human experiences, while the latter describes integration of your divinity.

The final initiation of the spiritual trinity (and the seven major centers of the body) is undoubtedly the most surprising because it involves returning to the place from which we've just ascended in an effort to manifest heaven on earth (Chapter 11). Some students and teachers have erroneously assumed that this initiation meant the completion of one's mission on earth and the next step on the path would, in effect, be to "ascend." This misunderstanding is often depicted by the mistaken imagery showing the spiritual energy of the body rising up the spine and out through the head. Although such a depiction is a valid form of "connecting with the cosmos" (as in some meditations), it cannot be overstated that nothing replaces the rarely taught significance of eventually channeling the energy that rises to the head, back down the front of the body. This process creates a complete circuit of energy, sometimes referred to as the microcosmic orbit. The concept of the energy of the body rising up the back and then being channeled down the front symbolizes the seventh and final initiation. It depicts the necessity of turning all spiritual beliefs into applicable experiences in our daily lives.

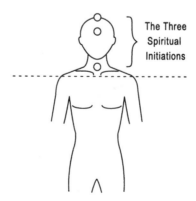

The Three
Spiritual
Initiations

9

Fifth Initiation:
The Spirit—Ether

The initiations and developmental stages of the fifth center of consciousness (which is also the first of the three spiritual centers and initiations) are the entryway back into the remembrance of our true divine self. The fifth center, or throat chakra, is sometimes referred to as the Christ center. We must all pass through this center because it acts as the "gates of heaven," which is why Jesus said, "No one will reach the Father but by me." (John 14:6) He was telling us that there is no way to merge with the Father–Mother God without remembering our role as the holy child.

The Christ center is symbolized by the fifth chakra on the body (counting upward from root to head) and by the five–pointed star, which heralded the birth of Jesus. The reverse of the Christ–star symbolism is found in the story of "the fall" of spirits from heaven. In scripture and mythology, Lucifer is referred to as the "fallen star" because he had forgotten who he really was. In fact, the Bible refers to all of us as "the stars that fell from heaven to the earth." (Revelation 6:13) However, when we move through lessons of awakening the inner Christ, we redeem ourselves and are placed back on the heavenly throne of divine awareness.

> *To practice the Presence of God is to awaken within us the Christ Consciousness. Christ is God in the soul of man. The resurrection is the death of the belief that we are separated from God.*
> —Ernest Holmes

A necessary lesson for attaining any level of Christ Consciousness is that *even* when you think you are trying to eliminate evil for the betterment of the world, as soon as you *identify* or judge something as evil, evil then exists. Instead, you are urged to learn to look at everything with spiritual objectivity and say, "Are you real (and expressing God's love), or are you unreal (and expressing fear)? Then, if it's real and of God, it will respond by shimmering with a brilliance greater than a thousand suns and will warm your heart with a sense of peace and acceptance. On the other hand, if it is not of God, then it does not exist in Reality and will disappear into the *nothing* that it is.

The initiation of Spirit involves the challenge to think and see as God does. For example, it's as if God is saying, "The thing that got you into this mess was the belief that you could separate, or be apart, from Me or that something might exist outside of My perfect love." To question the possibility of being separate from God—and even attempt to act it out—was a perfect test of your gift of free will. Now, the final "test" on the way home is to answer correctly the same question you didn't get right the first time, when you *seemed* to have parted ways with heaven: *Is there anything but God?* God is saying that if you want to pass this test and restore your divine awareness, you will gaze upon *everything* and ask if it is of Love *or* if it is of the fear that Love is not present. As soon as you decide there is anything but love, you are outside of Reality and experiencing the results of dreaming-up a separation from God and choosing to live on the dark side of the veil. However, if you choose to release judgments of good and evil and see things through divine eyes, you will experience an inner restoration. This transformational choice to see as God sees is not necessarily a one-time experience. Instead, it needs to be done on a consistent basis with all issues and questions that would draw you out of your center and bliss.

When observing the painful actions or experiences of others, without judging or becoming emotionally trapped, you will know that deep down what you are witnessing is a cry for love (and a call for healing) on the part of everyone involved. Your job, by analogy, is the same as if you were to see someone sinking in quicksand. You should offer a hand to pull the person out, but never jump in and sink with him or her.

At the Christ level of consciousness, you understand that to evaluate or judge a thing as evil and to say that it's the cause of your problems, actually magnifies its strength in the dream of separation. **The way a person, a war, or any personal crisis is transformed is NOT by praying to be saved *from* it, but rather by standing at the threshold of God and asking to see the problem through divine eyes.** Only then will you see the raving terrors of this world turned into the temporary cries for love they really are.

HOW IT LOOKS

In my personal life, I worked through the heart level and purging process that resulted in some powerful experiences and changes in my consciousness. Afterward, I had a dream that I was brought up to the fifth (and top) floor of a building, which symbolized the fifth initiation— the initiation of Christ Consciousness and my (our) connection with God.

Next, I was shown a dark, cloaked figure who, I was told, was the archetype of evil in the world—the being that caused every human woe. Then I was asked, "What will you choose to do with this evil?" My response was to pick up the evil being and prepare to throw it over the side of the building to destroy it—as a service to humanity. However, my guide said, "If you throw him to destroy him, you will *fail* the test." But, like most human beings, I thought that to destroy evil I had to do *something*, so I threw him anyway! I would later come to understand that our *judgment* of something as evil actually gives it life. Further, we cannot enter Christ Consciousness (or God Consciousness) with judgments weighing us down—no matter how seemingly justified.

ACCEPTING YOUR DIVINITY

There was a time when it was considered blasphemous to proclaim yourself as the Christ—or any such title, especially in the Western world. In fact, it's one of the main reasons that Jesus was crucified. Imagine a child of God who "wakes up" from the veil of illusion, realizes that he or she remains as originally created by God, feels ecstatic about this revelation, shares it with the world, and is therefore condemned to death. Thank God, we've come a long way—or have we?

Even today, most of us would hesitate to make such claims—especially in mixed religious company. Although there is something to be said for respecting other people's views and not making proclamations that would unnecessarily cause them to feel threatened, it should *never* be at the sacrifice of our connection to Truth. Of course, if we are *truly* connected to our Source, we won't feel the threat of being shaken in our convictions. However, **in our spiritual growth stages, we are temporarily more fragile and have to guard the inner Christ Child until it reaches maturity.**

All too often, when we *hesitate* to own our True Identity, we conveniently blame it on others for "keeping us bound" and "taking away our power." But remember that sitting across from a person who is *taking* away the power of another is usually a person who is *giving* it away. We are truly more afraid of our light than we are of our darkness. This fear explains why we allow the lesser force of our shadow self to exist. It's similar to the fact that we can more easily look at the moon than at the sun. By analogy, the moon is merely a reflection, or less intense version, of the sun (our Christ-Self, the sun/Son of God), which we believe is too overwhelming for us to view directly. Fortunately, this belief system is a dying one.

EVERY DAY IS CHRISTMAS

We live in the time of the Second Coming of Christ, and it is up to us to birth this Spirit within ourselves. Actually, we are experiencing this birthing process in large and small ways—daily and universally.

Two thousand years ago, the Essenes acted as midwives to the arrival of Christ in the flesh. Mary was pregnant with this Christ Child. Now, we are all pregnant with the Spirit of the Christ and can choose to celebrate the holy Christ-mass on a regular basis.

> *It is of utmost importance to every man that he experience within himself this "birth" of the Universal Christ. The universe is the body of Christ: everywhere present within it, without limitation, is the Christ Consciousness. If you expand your mind to receive Him, you will be blessed with the universal consciousness . . . Just as your consciousness pervades your whole body, the Consciousness of Christ is equally present throughout the cosmos — in every tree and plant, in every bird and animal, in every human being . . . Repeat this with me: "The vast consciousness of Christ is born this day within the cradle of my universal body, the cosmos. Unto me a child is given, unto me a child is born. I celebrate the birth of Christ in spirit and in body. The consciousness of Christ is all-pervading. Within the cradle of the universe, Christ and I are one."*
>
> — Paramahansa Yogananda

THE LIMITS OF SPIRIT

As all births have the potential of birth pains, so does the birth of our Christ self. This is not because pain is an aspect of the Christ but because **adapting to a new way of experiencing the world can have moments of disorientation.**

The initiation of Spirit is, in many respects, a renewal. So your body renews its cells, your nervous system gets rewired, and you feel a deeper sense of responsibility for the world. However, a challenging aspect of this new life is that it feels so good to experience, you may have mo-

ments of becoming *attached* to this blissful feeling. You may unconsciously decide to barely make a move, fearing you might *lose* this state
of being (which is the ego creeping in again!). However, this feeling of
uncertainty will eventually ease—especially with the help of the next
initiation, which is about permanent integration.

THE GIFTS OF THE SPIRIT

One of the most profound effects of feeling the presence of the Christ
Spirit is the attainment of true confidence. It's the sense of authority
that enabled Jesus to make comments such as, "I and my Father are one
and the same" (John 10:30) or "When you see me, you see the Father."
(John 14:9)

This Christlike level of consciousness underlies much of the phe-
nomenon often referred to as "the gifts of the Spirit" in various religious
traditions. It is the essence behind faith, true confidence, and an inner
knowingness because **true faith is not found at the level of human consciousness with its hope for the power of something
unseen. Rather, true faith rests in feeling connected to the
power of God and therefore *knowing* that all is well.** At this level
of awareness, it feels *right* and natural to have faith.

MODERN PARALLELS

In the Holy Grail legends, the Grail knight Percival finally passes his
initiations, finds the Grail (symbolic of attaining Christ Consciousness),
and returns it to the castle and its ruler, King Arthur. Then the land is
restored to its original fruitfulness. Similarly, when we pass our initiations and awaken the inner Christ, we reenter the Garden of Eden. The
deeper significance of the name Percival is now revealed. It means to
"pierce the veil" or destroy (pierce) evil. With the discovery of the Grail,
the veil that once separated humanity from the Christ/Divine Self (symbolized by the veil in Solomon's Temple) is now pierced, making the
way for Percival, and all who pass life's initiations to access and awaken
their inner Christ.

In *The Wizard of Oz*, Dorothy encounters the good fairy, who congratulates her for passing all of her initiations. She grants Dorothy (and her symbolic friends) everything that she sought. The fairy explains to Dorothy (and to us) that her ability to return home was with her all along. All she had to do was focus and affirm, "There's no place like home." We all know that, at the end of the story, Dorothy awakens to find that her adventure (evolutionary journey) was only a dream (illusion). She had been safely at home (in heaven) all along.

In *The NeverEnding Story*, the hero, Atreyu, passes his fifth initiation as he converses with a giant blue statue (conveniently the color of the fifth chakra). In this highly symbolic "children's movie," it is significant that before Atreyu reaches the Empress, he has to confront a beast who symbolizes evil. When Atreyu finally reaches the home of the Empress (symbolic of the sixth chakra), he completes his quest and saves Fantasia. All that he attains is experienced simultaneously within the consciousness of the little boy who is living the entire story in a parallel human existence. In the end, the beings that were destroyed by the evil forces are brought back to life, and some of these characters are then brought into the human boy's world (symbolizing the seventh initiation).

FACETS OF THE SPIRIT—ETHER

The three initiations of the spiritual states of consciousness can include lessons or studies related to the development of our Christ or Divine Self. To enhance your awareness of these spiritual facets of yourself, consider reading books related to inspiration, awakening your true self, and Christ Consciousness. You might also explore studies or practices such as mysticism, prayer, meditation, and communion with the higher realms.

Other ways to enhance your Christ Self include: colors—blues, purples, and translucent colors or shades; music—vocals, chanting, and gospel; instruments—flute and harp; gemstones—lapis, clear quartz crystal, amethyst, blue sapphire, and diamond.

FACETS OF THE THROAT CHAKRA

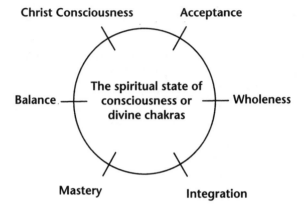

10

Sixth Initiation:
Integrating Life's Lessons

After reaching the fifth initiation and attaining a level of divine remembrance, sometimes referred to as Christ Consciousness, you would think the spiritual journey would be complete. But this is hardly the case. At this point, the journey of life is made far easier, partly because you now see through the illusions that used to control you. However, the sixth initiation (that of integration) calls you to absorb and integrate your divine identity, as well as to *become* the wisdom you've attained. This absorption, or integration process, is assisted by having the "down time" to breath in and contemplate your life's experiences. It's very similar to absorbing nutrients from the food and vitamins you ingest. Without absorbing the nutrients, the food or supplements are essentially worthless.

Lessons experienced but not learned will return. — **Anonymous**

In the life and initiations of Jesus, the scriptures tell us that after resisting the temptations in the desert, following His forty-day fast, Jesus was ministered to and comforted by angels. These are signs, or symptoms, of reaching the sixth initiation. Although it is sometimes a challenging period, the sixth initiation is often like reaching an oasis after a long desert journey. There is a reason for this respite. It's as though you are being prepared for the next leg of your journey—and you are. You'll soon realize that the journey continues.

> *Put off thy cares and thy clothes; so shall thy rest strengthen thy labor, and so thy labor sweeten thy rest.* — Francis Quarles

HOW IT LOOKS

In my own life, this sixth initiation mostly took the form of having a great deal of personal time for introspection. I wondered why my life seemed to have failed in so many ways and didn't dare bother trying to reconstruct a new life—certainly not when there was a chance of it all falling apart again! So, this was a time of great quiet. At first, it felt very awkward. But, eventually, I realized that this was my soul's way of doing a profound retrospection and meditation on life.

I realized that just as it is between lives, we reach the quietest moment of introspection before the dawn begins to break. Then a new calling draws us into the world again with renewed purpose. Feeling "born again," I would soon begin to hear a calling to continue my path as a healer and spiritual teacher—but at an entirely new, heightened level.

INNER PEACE BEFORE OUTER PEACE

A commonly overlooked sign of reaching a true sense of higher wisdom and integration is the ability to understand the difference between inner peace and outer peace. *Human consciousness* always looks to outside demonstrations for *external* proof of the peace that is sought (or for anything else prayed for). However, to possess *God Consciousness* means to experience a faith in the divine process even when there is no apparent reason. This is what led Jesus to say, "Blessed are those who have **not** seen and **still** believe." (John 20:29)

While humans express the need to see outer peace from war and other forms of conflict, Spirit knows that outer peace can be attained (and sustained) ONLY by achieving inner peace. In fact, those who have most integrated the concept of inner peace are able to smile in the face of adversity and pray for those who persecute them.

INTEGRATION MEANS IMMUNITY

Integration means to be or become the very thing that you study or learn. While you are still suffering from spiritual amnesia, you will feel like a victim in the world. Early on in the stages of awakening, you will learn how to protect yourself from negative, "outside" influences. But eventually you will learn that **in holding God's Presence as a part of your consciousness, you *are* only love, *attracting* only love, because there *is* only love.** Therefore, there is nothing to protect yourself from. This Reality will one day be learned and integrated by all—even if only one step at a time. On the other hand, if your frailty is such that you must avoid bad vibes or constantly protect yourself from people that you feel are beneath your level, then it is apparent that you have not truly integrated God's Presence into your being. God does not fear or avoid. **God Consciousness is not about avoidance of life's threats or issues, but rather immunity from them.** This immunity can only come from a real, integrated sense of love and acceptance for all beings.

THE DIVINE FEMININE

Now, while in the deep repose of the sixth initiation, it is not uncommon to experience a healing between you and your concepts of the supreme nurturer—the Divine Feminine. Here, you are held within the heart of God and feel a security, safety, and warmth that no human mother can provide. In fact, in your human experience, this is the very moment that you unconsciously long for and hold up as a standard of love that is impossible for any earthly woman to fulfill. Indeed, this blissful connection to the Divine Mother can be attained only by reaching the sixth initiation.

I am always within light, O Mother, always returning home to light. When these physical eyes close for the last time, darkness will dissolve into light, and light into you. —Ramprasad Sen

For some, the connection to the Divine Feminine is like a religious experience. For others, it's more like an energetic, alchemical fusion. In many arts of sacred sexuality, it is a primary goal to raise the life force from the lower energy centers of the body to the higher centers in the head that activate the pineal and pituitary glands. Here begins the victory dance of the god and goddess energies of ancient mythologies. **When the Divine Feminine is reawakened, it lovingly seduces the Divine Masculine, resulting in a new Creation. This new Creation ends up being a rebirth for you—one that you will experience in the next initiation, where heaven returns to earth once again.**

11

Seventh Initiation: Manifesting Heaven on Earth

The seventh, and final, initiation of life is also the third and final spiritual initiation. However, the word *final* does not actually mean the completion of our spiritual evolution as much as it indicates the end of a cycle. Once we complete this major cycle of spiritual initiations, we are asked to return to the earth plane, or our daily lives, to manifest a little more Light than there was a moment before. This situation is similar to what happens to many survivors of near death–experiences who describe being content to stay in such a heavenly space, yet are told to come back to finish their work on earth.

> *Be not merely good; be good for something*
> — Edgar Cayce (reading 279-1)

The workbook lessons found in *A Course in Miracles* offer great examples of how to choose an easier path in day-to-day life. These daily lessons take you through the whole process of retraining your mind to release old perceptions, followed by a period of disorientation and re-adjustment, and then refilling you with a new perspective on life. You end up experiencing a shift from the way you *thought* things *were* to the way God *knows* things *are*. It's a shift from human consciousness to the divine state of consciousness and experiencing heaven on earth. Ulti-mately, that's what the spiritual path is all about.

Once we've gone through a period of letting go of all of our past experiences and gifts, we find ourselves being called to pick them up again, or at least many of them. So now, when people need tarot card readings (for example) because that's what they believe in, then use tarot cards. If it's astrology they need, use astrology; if it's a hug, use a hug; if it's a thought, use a thought; if it's a massage, use a massage; and if it's silence they need, offer silence. You are now prepared to offer the gifts of God on an "as needed" basis and in whatever form will bring the most good for the most people. Even the experiences of your past that seemed less than divine are now transformed and have become valu-able tools to bring healing to the earth and all its inhabitants.

HOW IT LOOKS

My personal experience with this final initiation occurred when, af-ter basking in the bliss of a high level of spiritual presence, I was asked in a vision: "What has happened to all of your old tools and the things you learned?" I replied, "I left them all behind because now I'm *evolved* and don't need them anymore."

Spirit then said, "Go back, pick them up, and use them again." I wanted to ask, "Are you crazy? After all I went through to learn to let them go, you now want me to pick them up again?" Ohhhhh! I get it, I thought. This is a test to see if I am stupid enough to reinvest in the *worthless* tools of this world. But, no, the voice was quite serious and reassured me it was imperative that I now learn to reenter the world as a teacher and healer. However, this time I would be doing it differently.

In a way, God was telling me that I had to experience the letting go, so that I could gain a clearer understanding of my life and purpose. The final initiation, therefore, is about not only going back into the world, but following the spiritual path the easy way *instead* of the hard way. Now, there is far more *being* and less *doing*. There is more inspiration and insight and less struggle.

This level of initiation manifested as a vision that, in essence, told me, although I was enjoying the momentary respite of heaven's presence, it was time to return to my earthly life and work. As I previously said, for a moment, I actually thought this was a test of my intelligence. After all, who in their right mind, would choose to reenter the world of illusion that many lifetimes and initiations had taught them is meaningless? Yet, my Guide assured me this request was no joke and no test of my mental clarity. I was truly being encouraged to return to my old life and path. But now, I was to bring my *new self* to the world. I would no longer teach information I had merely learned or even believed. Instead, I was to teach what I *knew* and learn to live *as an integrated example*. My life has never been the same since.

GOD RECYCLES

This final initiation of manifesting heaven on earth is concealed in our esoteric anatomy and is seen symbolically in the human energy systems. For example, the kundalini energy rises up the back of the torso and, once it reaches the top of the head, flows down the front of the body. This descent is not a digression. In fact, it allows all that was achieved in the rising of energy to be integrated and brought back to the earthly realms for the greater good of all. This cycle is repeated until all lessons are learned and all has been transformed back into its original perfection.

In other words, the flow of our energy systems follows a course of evolution: upward to the greater heights of the spiritual centers, integration of these higher energies, and then back downward—but with a new level of consciousness. So, too, do we, as souls, follow a similar course. We descend into the material universe to experience human consciousness and learn our lessons, and then we ascend into higher realms and integrate what we have learned. Afterward, we return again to earth, but with a new, higher level of understanding.

WHY WE KEEP COMING BACK

Karma is like gravity—it keeps us bound to the earth. Yet, both laws are actually created by our collective souls as a self–governing discipline, more than they are (or were) "imposed by God." In other words, as the movie character Willie Wonka said, "We are the dreamers of the dream."

It is up to us to "anchor in" the Light and Love of God in the universe and in our own lives. Each transformation, large or small, in us (or in the world) occurs only when the perceptions in our hearts and souls are transformed. Through these shifts in consciousness, we are released from karma and discover the higher law of grace. Yet, **as long as there remains one illusion, opinion, judgment, or resentment held by any of us (consciously or unconsciously) about others or ourselves, we will continue to go through the cycles of rebirth and initiation until there is only love—as it was before the beginning of time.** We are the ones who choose! We are released (forgiven) as we release (forgive) others and surrender to learning the easy way.

ASCENDED MASTERS: THE EXCEPTION TO THE RULE

There are exceptions, however, to the karmic attraction to earth. **Once you attain a certain level of higher consciousness, returning becomes a choice rather than a necessity.** Although some souls might not choose to incarnate, they will most certainly continue to offer assistance to others on earth who are still undergoing their own initiations. The souls who reach this evolved level of consciousness are often referred to as "Ascended Masters." This term denotes a soul who has mastered enough of the material plane to *ascend* out of the evolutionary, initiatory cycle. Ascended Masters reach a point of lucidity within the dream of earthly life where they can choose to *incarnate* to offer assistance. They can also choose to remain outside the physical realm and simply reach down (from the higher realms) into the astral plane to assist others through whispered inspirations, nighttime dreams, and waking visions.

Yet, once again, for most souls, the journey of incarnating continues. After going through the various human initiations, we eventually attain a spiritual remembrance of our true self. Then, after reaching new levels of awareness, we are continually drawn into circumstances within the physical world to apply our remembrances (integrate them) and offer this new awareness to others—thus, manifesting heaven on earth.

Part V

The Journey Ends

Every soul who has ever lived has been a student of life's lessons and initiations and has been called to endure these sometimes challenging tests. Knowing this is what led Jesus (the Christ) to tenderly warn us all that the experience of awakening is like going out as "sheep among wolves." (Matthew 10:16)

As stated earlier, everyone is destined to go through the initiatory processes of the four human states of consciousness. After which, we will reach the *fifth initiation*—sometimes called the initiation of the Christ or the Second Coming. At this point, we have attained the first level of divine awareness. However, the *sixth initiation* calls us to integrate all that we've experienced during the five previous initiations. This sixth initiation, in part, is to prepare us for the *seventh spiritual initiation*, which is to discover ways to manifest our new awareness into the world for ourselves and others—thereby manifesting heaven on earth.

Before enlightenment: chopping wood, carrying water. After en-
lightenment: chopping wood, carrying water. — Zen **Proverb**

There is a great deal of irony to life's initiatory process. After we go to great lengths to "evolve" back into spiritual consciousness and away from the material world, **the final test lies in our ability to bring our renewed self back into the earth plane or make our spirituality a practical discipline.** The entire initiatory process can be eased and even shortened by knowing that, rather than waiting for the multistep process to be completed, we can live as though it were already complete. By bringing a heavenly state of self into the earth plane, we raise the level of consciousness and vibration closer to that of heaven—thus manifesting the prayer of Jesus, "Let Thy Kingdom come, on earth, as it is in heaven." (Matthew 6:10)

You might often wonder what is the purpose of all of these complicated processes, cycles, and experiences. Why did you choose these lessons in the first place? Why didn't you wake up sooner, and why did you resist your awakening so persistently? Yet, in the end, when you see what new attainments come to you (after being so patient and vigilant with these initiations of life), you will feel a humble sense of gratitude. You will focus less on what could have been and more on what truly was and is. This is especially true when you witness, firsthand, the effects your transformed self can have on the life of another soul (or souls) who may be struggling with something that you have already cycled through.

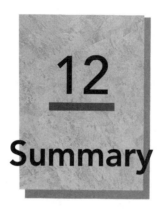

12

Summary

IN THE END, THERE IS A PURPOSE AFTER ALL

Completing a major cycle of initiations is like reaching a new, higher level of spiritual maturity and awareness. The process is not unlike raising a child. You go through a period of struggle and conflict as that child resists the call and need for healthy boundaries. Also, like a parent raising a child, you might become disheartened during this natural growth process. Yet, the day usually comes when you see how your love and persistence has paid off. Of course, parenting, like large–scale initiations, is made easier when you let go of your personal agendas.

So what is the payoff for enduring life's challenges and initiations? In essence, you feel more whole and complete, as well as free and at peace. You now recognize your part in learning to gain new perspectives of yourself and the world around you. You see everyone and everything in a new light. You begin to master more of the states of human consciousness (and their numerous facets), as well as integrating more Divine Consciousness. You resist life's lessons less often and learn to see trials as your own misperceptions being called to transformation, knowing something better awaits—the dawning of a new day.

Another major awareness that results from consciously walking through our initiations is that even when we keep our focus on the truth of who we are, we will still encounter lessons, cycles, and phases of growth or remembrance. In fact, **we learn to measure our growth process not by having an absence of challenges, but by the ability to recognize when we slip, as well as choosing to bounce back quickly (regaining our balance).** Nevertheless, until the moment of "total awakening," we can expect to have smaller awakenings along the way—in our dreams, visions, and in other forms as well. In fact, there is an extraordinary similarity between birth, dreams, death, meditation, and spiritual visions. First of all, they all include a shift from one reality or state of consciousness into another. They all involve the gift of messages and/or lessons, and they often meet with occasional resistance. They also teach us how temporary each stage of life can be, since we always wake up into a different reality.

CONCLUSION

When all lessons are learned, we are able to see that behind them all were our own false beliefs. Although at our deepest core lies a perfect spark of God's presence, this was heavily masked over by our own patterns of limitation and belief systems (sometimes personified as the ego), which then acted as a god who began creating our world and attracting our lessons and experiences. We now realize that our evolutionary experiences were never really about God sending us forth to learn something new or gather information. It was never God telling us we had debts to pay or perfection to achieve. It was always about us! We only learned lessons that *we* thought we had to learn, paid debts that *we* thought we owed, and collected debts that *we* thought others owed us. The final awakening (which only occurs after numerous smaller awakenings) is a liberation from all of these opinions, illusions, and false beliefs. It's a release from all beliefs other than God's and a surrendering of our opinions to God's perfect knowingness.

The universe is a school where people will eventually develop into the image and likeness of God. It will exist as long as a school is needed. — Peace Pilgrim

The end of the soul's journey is much the same—just another shift in perception. It's simply the final "curtain call." Just as the body has its moment of death when its mission is complete, so does the soul eventually surrender its existence and ascend back into Spirit. At that moment, the Spirit awakens to a level of awareness where there are no more lessons to learn. Then, there is a realization that the soul was only sleeping and dreaming of a world of fear and separation and is now awake in the mind and heart of God.

The purpose of the seven initiations on the spiritual path can be summarized in three stages. First, (Initiations One–Three) you experience something in your life involving a person, object, emotion, event, or thought. Second, (Initiation Four) your soul finds ways to get you to integrate a meaning from that experience—a new understanding that will in some way expand your consciousness. Third, (Initiation Five–Seven) you will gather whatever meaning you have integrated from your experience and then send out creative thoughts to inform the universe of your new level of understanding.

If you have learned well and allowed the previous experience to raise your consciousness, you will see a brighter future—one that involves healing and/or new, fresh beginnings. On the other hand, if you resist or deny the lessons in each experience, your soul will bring forth harder lessons that are less likely to be missed. Every event in your life arose from this three-stage process and continues as long as you are part of earth's evolutionary cycles.

Once you truly understand this evolutionary process as a cycle created by you, it's much easier to see that you are a co-creator of your life and of the universe at large. You will then understand how **your actions, decisions, and responses of yesterday attracted what you are experiencing today; and the decisions of today affect what you create for tomorrow.**

ABOUT MICHAEL MIRDAD

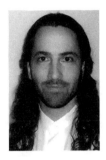

Michael Mirdad, spiritual teacher, author, and intuitive healer, has an extensive background in spirituality, parapsychology, and metaphysics and has taught in the largest metaphysical schools in the world for over twenty years. He has facilitated thousands of classes, lectures, workshops, and private sessions throughout the world. Michael is noted in such books as *Initiation Into Miracles* by Nigel Taylor. He also guides advanced students on yearly journeys to sacred sites around the world (such as Greece, Egypt, Great Britain, France, and the Yucatan) where he also conducts workshops.

Dr. Mirdad is respected as one of the finest and most diverse spiritual teachers and healers of our time by numerous authors, students, and masters. He is especially noted for his visionary ability to bring forth the highest Truths and spiritual principles and present them in a concise, applicable manner. Michael Mirdad has also acted as spiritual consultant and advisor on motion pictures.

Michael Mirdad may be reached at: Grail Productions, P.O. Box 2783, Bellingham, WA 98227. Visit his web site at www.grailproductions.com or contact him at 360-671-8349 or grailpro@aol.com.

DISCOVER HOW THE EDGAR CAYCE MATERIAL CAN HELP YOU!

The Association for Research and Enlightenment, Inc. (A.R.E.®), was founded in 1931 by Edgar Cayce. Its international headquarters are in Virginia Beach, Virginia, where thousands of visitors come year-round. Many more are helped and inspired by A.R.E.'s local activities in their own hometowns or by contact via mail (and now the Internet!) with A.R.E. headquarters.

People from all walks of life, all around the world, have discovered meaningful and life-transforming insights in the A.R.E. programs and materials, which focus on such areas as personal spirituality, holistic health, dreams, family life, finding your best vocation, reincarnation, ESP, meditation, and soul growth in small-group settings. Call us today at our toll-free number:

1-800-333-4499

or

Explore our electronic visitors center on the
Internet: **http://www.edgarcayce.org.**

We'll be happy to tell you more about how the work of the A.R.E. can help you!

A.R.E.
215 67th Street
Virginia Beach, VA 23451-2061